Pathology of eating

Social and Psychological Aspects of Medical Practice

Editor: Trevor Silverstone

Pathology of eating

Psychology and treatment

Sara Gilbert, BA, MSc

Senior Clinical Psychologist
Northwick Park Hospital, Harrow

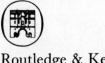

Routledge & Kegan Paul
London and New York

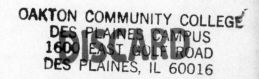

First published in 1986 by
Routledge & Kegan Paul Ltd
11 New Fetter Lane, London EC4P 4EE

Published in the USA by
Routledge & Kegan Paul Inc.
in association with Methuen Inc.
29 West 35th Street, New York, NY 10001

Set in 11 on 12 pt Imprint
by Inforum Ltd, Portsmouth
and printed in Great Britain
by St Edmundsbury Press Ltd
Bury St Edmunds, Suffolk

Library of Congress Cataloging in Publication Data

Gilbert, Sara D.
Pathology of eating.
(Social and psychological aspects of medical practice)
Bibliography p.
Includes index.
1. Appetite disorders. 2. Psychotherapy. I. Title. II. Series
DNLM: 1. Appetite Disorders – etiology. 2. Appetite Disorders –
therapy. WM 175   9466p
RC552.A72G65   1986   016.85'2   86–6608

British Library CIP Data also available
ISBN 0–7102–0271–7

Contents

Acknowledgments

I should like to thank Mrs Sheila Bramson for her permission to reproduce the poem on page 92–3.

I am grateful to Mrs Jennifer Frampton and all the library staff at the Clinical Research Centre for their painstaking help with literature searches and with tracing references.

My thanks go also to Mrs Christine Hawkins for her help with the typing of the manuscript.

Preface

Overeating and undereating are phenomena which in the past decade have captured the interest and imagination of health professionals and public alike.

The definition of overeating and undereating in itself poses a dilemma, coloured by subjectivity and bound by culture. A part of the problem is the separation of weight characteristics from assumptions about behaviour. Moreover the kinds of food eaten on different occasions and by different people vary from one culture to another. Even within societies, what may comprise a normal amount of food on one day may be seen as abnormal on the next. The situation is complicated by our inadequate understanding of what triggers eating, and what indicates to us that it is time to stop. Some of the crucial elements may be very different for different people, and psychological factors such as perceived time of day, thoughts about food, or the range of foods available, may all have powerful, if hidden effects on the amount we eat at any one time.

Psychological treatments for overeating and undereating are drawn from several different theories about causation. The link between aetiological theory and therapeutic practice is in some instances readily apparent, but in others almost non-existent. Moreover understanding is complicated by the frequent use of the same term to describe different therapies: for example the terms 'psychotherapy' and 'behaviour therapy' rarely denote uniformity of technique or of approach across studies, or when applied across a range of disorders.

In Part I of this book, an attempt will be made to describe normal eating behaviour, taking into account the constraints of cultural difference.

In Part II of the book, overeating and undereating will

be described, in the context of people of normal weight as well as in relation to people who are underweight or overweight. Emphasis will be placed on the psychological aspects of overeating and undereating, both in relation to systemic disease and in relation to social-psychological or psychiatric phenomena and the problems of clarifying the interface between them and identifying causes.

In Part III of the book, treatments for overeating and undereating will be outlined, again with the emphasis on psychological methods and the psychological effects of treatment itself.

Part I

Normal eating behaviour

Cultural aspects of eating and body weight

1

The kind of food we eat and the style in which we eat it is an essential part of the fabric of society. There are some genetic biases determining what we take or reject as food; but for most people eating the correct amount and balance of nutrients is no purely automatic process like the ability to breathe. On the contrary what we eat is to a large extent determined by cultural, social and psychological pressures (Rozin, 1982). The culture into which a person is born, for example, determines the availability and limits of what there is to eat. It determines what food is appropriate to eat and what is not. For example, the use or avoidance of particular animal foods are often ethnic and religious markers (Simoons, 1982). A universal influence on the food habits of many races is that of religious dietary laws, which restrict what is eaten, how, when and with whom. In addition, certain foods may become the symbol of national culture. Rozin (1976) has suggested that the particular cuisine of a culturally coherent group serves as one of many ways of identifying that group, setting it apart from other groups, and also of making social distinctions within members of the group. In India the caste system not only determines the type of food to be eaten or not but also with whom one can eat and by whom the food must and must not be prepared (Carlson *et al.*, 1984).

Food is also in a sense, then, a means to communicate with other people. Hence we eat certain foods on particular occasions – on festivals, birthdays, celebrations. On other occasions we may abstain from some foods, or not eat at all as on religious fast-days. We may communicate our interests in, respect for or friendship towards colleagues, visitors or friends, by sharing a meal with them. In the Western world a meal in one's home has connotations which are different from those of taking a meal in a restaurant. In all cultures to eat alone has a very different meaning from that of eating with another person. Particular meals often have largely ritual value: for example the wedding breakfast, Christmas lunch, the Jewish Passover supper, the ritual of 'eating together' practised by the Cêwa tribe in East Africa as a sign of attachment (Marwick, 1965); these meals have less to do with the need to fuel the body than with the practice of long-held traditions and the symbolic representation of special relationships. In the same way to eat too much or too little often conveys a message to other people – consider for example the emotional impact of the hunger strike.

The consequences of eating include short- and long-term physiological effects – taste, fullness, long-term health or disease; but there is a case for the notion that much of what we learn about the effects of specific foods is mediated by cultural influences (Rozin and Fallon, 1981). Such influences may include what we are told about the health-giving properties of foods, and their social meaning – for example caviare and wine are for the rich and cultured, berries of a certain type are dangerous.

There are also historical aspects to the amount and types of food that we eat. To a large extent this is determined by availability and by wealth as much as by individual preferences. There is a widely held assumption that most 'normal' people will eat only as much as they need, given food in plentiful supply. Yet literature abounds with prosaic descriptions of meals throughout the ages from the Bible to the present day, and civilised man has always been tempted to eat more than enough. Suetonius has been quoted as saying that the downfall of the Roman empire was due to the apathy and gluttony of the people. The Emperor Augustus even tried to limit the amount of food bought by limiting the expenditure allowed on certain meals (Fitzgibbon, 1981).

Not only is man able to eat more than he needs, but his choice of food and the way in which nutrients are combined may vary from social group to social group and from generation to generation depending on social and economic circumstances. Within what we commonly know as Western society alone, approximately 25 per cent of household expenditure goes on food and this may vary by as much as 20–30 per cent according to level of income (McKenzie, 1980). If people vary their diet according to economic circumstances, this will have a large

4

effect particularly on the consumption of fresh foods such as fruit, meat, and fish.

More fundamental changes in eating habits occur as people move from the culture of pre-industrial societies to that of the West. The sad casualties of this transitional stage are living proof of the fact that the knowledge of what is good for us to eat is determined less by inborn genetic influences than by social and cognitive factors. For example on the island of Nauru in the Pacific, the traditional meal pattern has been replaced by one of irregular snacking of foods high in carbohydrates throughout the day and the very high incidence of diabetes is far greater than that in other Pacific islands with a less Westernised life-style (Hankin *et al.*, 1970, cited by Freimer *et al.*, 1983). The phenomenon of so-called acculturation illustrates the way in which patterns of food intake can follow fashions, albeit often in a less extreme manner. For example in Britain in the 1970s consumption of cakes and pastries went down by 38 per cent while those of ice-cream, mousse and soufflé nearly doubled (King, 1983). Meanwhile, an increasing number of meals taken outside the home could be defined as 'snacks' rather than 'main meals', and a steadily higher proportion of food eaten derives its energy from fat and animal protein at the expense of carbohydrate (King, 1983).

In the Western world in particular, there are three major influences on current patterns of food intake that differentiate us from previous societies. One of these is that adequate if not abundant supplies of food are available to more people than ever before. The second is that most food items can now be bought cooked, packaged and ready to eat so that we no longer have complete control over the ingredients used to prepare them. The third is that at the same time we have become more sedentary than ever before, so that ironically we may be growing increasingly economical in our use of the abundant food that is available (Cannon and Einzig, 1983).

In this context, it is perhaps not surprising that obesity has become one of the largest health problems of our time. In England alone, 31 per cent of men and 27 per cent of women are at least 10 per cent above acceptable weight (Report of the Royal College of Physicians on Obesity, 1983). It is true to say that not all obese people eat more than slim people do, but if all that is required to become obese is an intake of food greater than

5

necessary to maintain energy balance, then the existence of a surfeit of palatable foods, often of illusory nutritional value, and coupled with a decreasing need to expend energy must have a part to play in weight gain for at least some obese people.

Whatever the reality of the relationship between body weight and eating behaviour, still the relationship is generally assumed to be a direct one and to communicate to other people something not only about the eating habits but also about the personality and even the social status of the person concerned.

In the underdeveloped countries of the world obesity is rare, especially in poor communities. Here to be obese is a sign of relative wealth. As such, obesity is admired as a sign of fertility, strength and prosperity (Garner et al., 1983). Fatness is also a sign of beauty in some cultures, and among African tribes the practice of sending young women to fattening houses in preparation for marriage is still common today (Ley, 1980). In the Western world too, for a woman to be plump was considered a sign of beauty until this century. This is now no longer the case however, and the relationship of obesity with class has also changed. There is a sharp contrast between the relationship of obesity to social class in the cities of the Western world and in the less affluent societies of Central America, South China and India. Studies in both New York and London have suggested that obesity is far more prevalent in the lower socio-economic classes than in the upper social classes and that this relationship is particularly true for women (Moore et al., 1962; Silverstone et al., 1969; Garn et al., 1977).

One possible factor contributing to this phenomenon is the difference in the quality of foods affordable by people of different classes. Another factor likely to contribute is that of the attitudes of other people to obese people and the effect of this on the obese person's potential for upward social mobility.

Prejudice against people who are overweight is well-established. Many studies with children and adults, professionals and non-professionals alike, have yielded the same conclusion. In relation to children, methods have included showing line drawings of children of different body shape, or photographs of obese, thin or deformed children. These studies have suggested that children consistently rate pictures of obese children as less liked than pictures of normal weight or thin children (Lerner and Gellert, 1969). Pictures of fat children evoke descriptions such as 'cheats', 'sloppy', 'naughty', 'stupid', 'dirty' even at an early age (Staffieri, 1967). In another study pictures of obese children were rated less likeable than drawings not only of normal-looking children but of children with physical deformities such as a missing left hand, or a facial disfigurement (Richardson *et al.*, 1961).

Children are not alone in their prejudice. In a study which replicated that of Richardson and his colleagues (1961), Maddox (1968) selected groups of males and females, black and white, college educated and high school educated, as well as a predominantly lower status medical outpatient clinic population. All the groups, including the overweight people themselves, rated the overweight child as the least likeable. Other negative characteristics have also been attributed to obese people. For example they were placed at the low evaluative ends of scales such as 'attractive', 'old', 'successful', 'influential', 'follower', and less likely than other people to be wives or sisters (Chetwynd *et al.*, 1975). These attitudes figure also in the behaviour of people towards the obese. For example, people are less likely to comply with a request from an obese person than from a thin person (Steinberg and Birk, 1983). Students may be less likely to be accepted for university education if they are obese (Canning and Mayer, 1966), despite the fact that people who are fat are no less intelligent than people of normal weight. The obese are discriminated against at work too, and are less likely to be employed than are thin people of equivalent ability. At the executive level they often earn less than do their thin counterparts (studies cited in Wadden and Stunkard, 1985). Even among the helping professions attitudes toward the obese are no less negative. A group of rehabilitation counselling students was shown pictures of male and female 'clients' of different weights but with the same history attached to the pictures. The students had to say what they thought the most likely outcome would be for the 'clients' and choose service delivery options for them. The massively obese women were rated more negatively than both the normal weight males and the normal weight females on counsellor feelings. When given identical information, the students had more positive attitudes towards a 'client' who was shown as normal weight than to one shown as obese. Moreover when portrayed as obese, the 'client' was more likely to be recommended for adjustment services (counselling, a sheltered workshop) and less likely to be funded for college training.

The obese are seen as eating more than people of average weight (Harris, 1983), and as having 'no will power' (Maiman *et al.*, 1979) by students and professionals respectively. In summary, obese people are seen by others, including the obese themselves, as less worthy of respect than are other people. They are assumed to have brought the condition upon themselves through overeating; gluttony implies sinfulness and indeed the obese may be seen in as negative a light as offenders (Homant and Kennedy, 1982).

The negative attitude to the obese appears to be particularly strong in relation to women.

The pressure for people to be slim, and women in particular, is reflected everywhere in the media. One has only to glance at the advertisements on the television to notice that the mother who uses the gentlest washing-up liquid, the girlfriend of the man who has bought the new car, the girl who accepts a box of special chocolates, all are slim. A survey of body types portrayed on the television carried out in 1978 bears this out (Kurman, 1978, cited by Garner *et al.*, 1983). Less than 2 per cent of the actors were obese; and youth, the female sex and positive personality attributes were all related to thinness. The caricature of the fat person as the stupid, the interfering, the person not to be taken seriously, appears to figure strongly in the media. It is no longer fashionable, although acceptable, even for opera singers to be fat.

Wooley and Wooley (1979) have reviewed studies relating to society's attitude towards the obese and conclude that from adolescence onward, females are more greatly affected than males by the climate of prejudice against fatness. The pressure for women in particular to be slim is reflected in the content of magazines both for men and for women. Garner *et al.* (1980) studied the pictures of *Playboy* magazine centre page girls and of the winners of the 'Miss America pageant' from 1959 to 1978 and found that the ideal shapes for women became increasingly thinner over the years. The number of magazines and books devoted to slimming and diet foods has rapidly increased in the last ten years alone. The proportion of space given to material about diet and slimming in six major women's magazines was shown to increase significantly during the ten years between

1969 and 1979 compared with the previous ten years (Garner *et al.*, 1980). During the same period the authors state that the average weight of women under the age of thirty was consistently several pounds heavier in 1979 than in 1959. In other words the increasingly slim images portrayed in the media are not representative of the actual size of the average woman today.

Thus, the average weight of both men and women is increasing; but at the same time the pressure to be slim is growing and particularly in relation to women. Fatness is perceived in a negative light and in order to be loved, admired and respected it is important to be slim. These conflicting pressures coincide with increased affluence and the increasing availability of an ever larger variety of foods, both easily prepared and ready to eat. It has been suggested that the exhortation to eat vegetables and to diet now universal in Euro-American culture contrasts strongly with the contradictory habit of marketing high fat, high sugar, high calorie, high salt and low fibre foods as rewards; that in our attempt to save the situation we have become compulsive, even unrealistic, in the extent to which we now advocate dieting and exercise (Mackenzie, 1985).

In this climate it is thought by many people that large numbers of women are more predisposed than ever before to the development of eating disorders, in particular anorexia nervosa and bulimia. Certainly there is an increasing number of women of normal weight who profess to be currently overweight and who are attempting to diet, for much of the time. In survey of college students, a far larger proportion of students believes itself to be overweight than that which is actually overweight (Halmi *et al.*, 1981). At the same time there are many women who are involved in an ongoing battle for control of their weight. In a survey in Manhattan more than 60 per cent of 166 college women admitted to having spent some time dieting during the past school year, based on information gained largely from newspapers and magazines; but only 9 per cent of these women were actually obese (Grunewald, 1985). For other women the problems go further than just those of keeping to the latest popular diet and there is evidence that some 20 per cent of young women may have problems with binge-eating from time to time.

It has been suggested that a constant struggle for control of their weight may for some women have come to represent a more fundamental struggle for the control of their lives in general, in a society which sets impossible standards for perfection. Hence the ability to diet and stay thin becomes an outward sign to the rest of the world that the woman is in control, even if the appearance is maintained by alternate bingeing and purging, while the person who remains fat may convey the message that on the one hand she is out of control, while on the other that she is a rebel and not prepared to succumb to the expectations of a society that puts unreasonable demands for perfection on its female members.

Being overweight and on a diet, or maintaining an unnaturally slim figure by starving also entitle many women to membership of certain clubs. The person who is on a diet feels a certain affinity with other people who are suffering the same deprivations.

Many slimming clubs carry the analogy of overeating with sinning through in their meetings; they are likened by observers to churches where people can join with others to confess their transgressions and to worship the ideals of slimness and abstention (Allon, 1975; Cannon and Einzig, 1983). More recently, the Women's Movement in both the United States and England has taken on the issue of body weight and eating in relation to feminism, and the religion of strict dieting has been replaced for many people by the attempt to join with others to become more aware of themselves and their role in relation to society.

There are of course situations where overeating or undereating arise as symptoms of disease. Often the first sign of an illness may be unwillingness or inability to eat resulting in weight loss which alerts other people to the problem. However undereating and overeating have also become phenomena which are symptomatic of certain relationships – between individuals, within families, and as vehicles for a special kind of affinity within social groups. A major part of the modern dilemma is in establishing a definition of where disease ends and a phenomenon of culture and modern society begins.

The control of feeding and weight

2

There is a common assumption that eating in response to hunger is a function akin to filling the petrol tank of one's car in preparation for a long journey. However the science of food-intake is complex and the nature of what is involved still poorly understood. It is possible to eat when 'full' and to choose not to eat when empty, but at the same time most people maintain a fairly constant weight in the short term and in the longer term weight fluctuates by only about ten kilograms (Garrow, 1978).

Several different phenomena have been studied in attempts to tease out exactly how intake and weight are controlled. These include internal physiological factors on the one hand; and external, environmental factors such as the palatability of the food available and the social and cultural context on the other. As always where the subjects of research are human, the findings are complicated by psychological phenomena – the experience and expectations of the people concerned; yet there is no cut and dried division between the purely physiological and the purely psychological.

Many physiological factors have been suggested as contributors to feeding behaviour. Stomach contractions are the most obvious possibility in relation to the popular view of hunger, but even complete removal of the innervation of the stomach itself has no effect on the experience of hunger or on the control of intake (Garg and Singh, 1983). The level of sugar in the blood, caloric regulation through the stomach, and stomach distension all appear to have an effect on the amount eaten by animals and man, but these do not necessarily imply regulation based on direct signals from the local areas themselves.

Brain mechanisms

The search for central mechanisms regulating intake has continued for many years. It might at first be tempting to assume a simple system like that which exists in the fly. The fly's feeding behaviour has been described by Hernandez and Hoebel (1980) as a 'thermostat'; when deprived of food for some time, the fly's taste and gastric receptors fire, and carry on firing until the fly is full up. If the neural connections between the gut and central mechanism are severed, the fly will continue to eat until it bursts. In man, however, gastric distention on its own is certainly no adequate indicator of readiness to stop eating, for the mechanisms which tell us whether we are food-deprived or not are more complex both in themselves, and in their susceptibility to influence from other sources.

Nevertheless, in the early part of this century, the existence of several clinical cases in which tumours of the hypothalamus were associated with obesity contributed to the idea that in man, too, there is one satiety and feeding centre in the brain (Balagura, 1972). Much of the research into feeding behaviour in vertebrates has since then centred around the hypothalamus which is considered to be the site of mechanisms controlling energy balance and the motivation to eat. Experiments designed to investigate its functioning have used a variety of methods, including brain lesions, electrical stimulation, recording from single neurons, and neuropharmacological manipulations.

Interest in the hypothalamus began in 1940, when Hetherington and Ransom showed that lesions in the ventromedial hypothalamus of the rat resulted in overeating or hyperphagia leading to obesity. Anand and Brobeck (1951) subsequently discovered that lesions in the lateral hypothalamus led to a failure to eat, or aphagia, and a failure to drink, adypsia. Similarly, other studies showed that electrical stimulation of the lateral hypothalamus led to eating; and of the ventromedial hypothalamus to cessation of eating. Studies of this type led in the 1950s and 1960s to the 'dual centre' hypothesis: the view that food intake is regulated by a feeding centre in the lateral hypothalamus, and a reciprocally acting satiety centre in the ventromedial nucleus of the hypothalamus.

More recent findings have led to some modifications of the

theory (Grossman, 1976). For example the lesions can be shown to produce gross sensory and motor disturbances which may themselves produce changes in eating behaviour. Thus lesions of the ventromedial nucleus of the hypothalamus produce metabolic disturbances that cause overeating indirectly through increased removal of essential fuels from circulation. Also the lesions themselves produce sensory enhancement and animals with these lesions will overeat only when the food is highly palatable. Incidentally this suggests that satiety is a relative phenomenon influenced by hedonic as well as by purely physiological factors (Grossman, 1984). Animals with lateral hypothalamic lesions on the other hand show sensory neglect of touch, odour and taste. They also become apathetic, and hence cannot be bothered to eat but in fact may do so again after recovery from the lesion or can be stimulated to do so with the help of amphetamines or having their tails pinched! Up to 40 or 60 per cent of the effects on eating may be due in part also to the effects on other fibres such as those of the nigrostriatal tract, resulting in depletion of striatal dopamine. Recent neurochemical data have identified specific chemical pathways in the brain which suggest a role for catecholamine systems in feeding which does not necessitate the physical existence of satiety and hunger 'centres' *per se* (Blundell, 1980). Nevertheless, while the hypothalamus is no longer considered to be largely a centre which sends out signals to eat and not to eat, it is now seen as integrating many sensory and metabolic factors. These include a major peripheral input from adipose tissue, from gut hormones, and from receptors in the gasto-intestinal tract (Stellar, 1984).

Set-point theory

Weight is maintained at a fairly constant level whether high or low; this is not fully explained by the idea of hypothalamic regulation as even animals with hypothalamic damage maintain a constant, albeit very low or very high weight. A theory which attempts to explain this phenomenon revolves around the idea that there is a biological 'set-point' to weight (Nisbett, 1972). The theory has its basis in the fact that within individuals weight remains fairly stable over long periods of time. If weight is lost, metabolic rate drops to a proportionately greater degree and if weight is gained, metabolic rate goes up more than would be predicted from the increase (Keesey and Corbett, 1984). Therefore when people become obese, the mechanism which should operate in this way to make them lose weight appears to have failed. Set-point theory holds that on the contrary the mechanism has simply been set at a higher level to maintain abnormally high body weights in obese people. The theory draws on evidence from the animal literature for its support. For example animals with lesions of the hypothalamus do not recover their lost weight but maintain their weight at the new lower level as precisely as they did at the previous level; they defend this weight as well as do normal weight animals even in the face of forced-feeding or tricks designed to make them eat more (Keesey *et al.*, 1976). In addition at the other end of the spectrum the weights of obese Zucker fatty rats are also maintained at consistent levels even in the face of caloric trickery. Set-point theory postulates that some humans similarly have a high number of fat cells and so are bound to maintain a high weight whatever their circumstances or however they might try to push their weight down.

The theory is difficult to prove conclusively however as it is impossible to discern whether people maintain a high body weight because they are programmed to do so or whether they are simply eating more than their neighbours in response to the many temptations which exist in the environment.

Hunger and satiety

The investigation of short-term control of feeding is a somewhat less problematic area than the investigation of long-term regulation if only because experiments can be set up which have a beginning and an end within a fairly convenient period of time. Since eating is popularly held to be triggered by 'hunger' and stopped when a state known as 'satiety' is reached, these two phenomena have frequently been taken as independent variables in research on the control of food intake.

Both states are difficult to define as they are largely subjective in nature. The term 'hunger' is usually assumed to represent a physiological need for food while 'appetite', representative rather of desire without necessarily a physiological basis, is more ambiguous. The difficulty is that neither is an observable state.

'Satiety' represents the 'zone' (Van Itallie and Vanderweele, 1981) between that state in which hunger, although not necessarily appetite, is absent, and that in which discomfort or overfullness are experienced.

There are two interrelated components to satiety: intermeal satiety, which determines the length of time between meals, and intrameal satiety which may determine the speed at which food is eaten (Van Itallie and Vanderweele, 1981). There is no clear mechanism for triggering eating and most of what we do know relates rather to what makes us stop at the end of a meal. Pregastric components such as taste and smell, gastric and intestinal receptors, levels of circulating glucose and changes in hormone concentrations may all have a part to play in determining satiety. What little is known about the physiology of satiety has been described elsewhere (Smith, 1982), but if physiological cues do exist, the evidence is that we do not always heed them, and that they may be overriden. One fairly plausible explanation of this phenomenon is that sensations which trigger satiety for one person are different in degree from those which signal satiety for another; in that, for example, some individuals claim to enjoy the feeling of being 'full-up' to the point almost of discomfort while others prefer not to experience even the slightest distension after a meal. At the same time, however, there are other, hidden, factors at work which appear to act on the experience of satiety itself.

Factors affecting satiety and our choice of food

Calories versus taste or appearance

It is tempting to imagine that physiological control of what we eat is so sensitive that we must automatically 'know' when we have taken enough calories in food whatever its composition, and however unfamiliar it may be. This idea has been questioned many times in studies involving the use of preloads. The subjects of these studies are sometimes patients kept in hospital with the aim of losing weight, or, more often, undergraduate students at university. They are given food or drink in disguised form prior to a test meal and the amount consumed in this meal is subsequently measured. The preload may take the form of a drink, or a soup, the calorific value of which can be altered without necessarily altering the taste or texture. In experiments such as these, the results suggest that altering the calorific value of a preload has little effect on how many calories are eaten subsequently; in other words, people do not necessarily respond to the nutritive value of what they have just eaten by eating more or less immediately afterwards.

They do, however, sometimes eat differently in response to the appearance or taste of what they have just eaten. We may eat less after a drink designed to appear high in calories than after the same drink designed to appear low in calories (Wooley, 1972). Similarly we may eat less after something we perceive as sweet than after something perceived as not so sweet, whether it was high or low in calories (Brala and Hagen, 1983).

A criticism of this kind of experiment is that it is very short-term, usually spanning only a few hours. We regulate our weight over long periods of time, and so it is feasible that if we are 'fooled' on Monday into eating more or less, we may make up for it by Friday, or even by several Mondays hence. There is in fact some evidence that people do regulate their eating over time to counter-balance the effects of varying preloads, but that the amount by which they regulate does not necessarily match exactly the preload differences (Spiegel, 1973; Durrant *et al.*, 1982).

These considerations do not detract however from the possibility that in the short term at least, physiological mechanisms are linked closely with cognitive ones. In other words the effects of feeling, tasting and ingesting food are tempered by those of seeing, smelling, learning about and thinking about food. It is common knowledge that the sight, smell, and even the thought of food can itself bring on an appetite which is indistinguishable from the hunger produced by prolonged deprivation, and if we can be fooled by undergraduate experiments then how much greater must be the possibilities afforded by the hard-sell, fast food environment of the civilised world?

Palatability

Foods have different levels of palatability for different people. This is clear from the point of view of preferences even within families; preferences vary between cultures, exemplified by the diverse range of culinary styles available in the high street. Several experimenters investigating effects on eating have varied the palatability of food offered to people, sometimes by their own definition of what is palatable and sometimes by taking into account individual preferences. The more palatable the food, the more people will eat (Hill and McCutcheon, 1975) and the more quickly they will eat it! (Bellisle and le Magnen, 1981). The importance of palatability is fairly clear also from some of the earlier experiments which were designed to investigate aspects of energy balance. In these experiments less attention was given to the taste properties of the food than to its calorific value. The easiest way of measuring intake is to provide a food of uniform nature; hence in an experiment where subjects had to feed themselves a uniform tasting liquid nutrient through a food dispenser over several days they not surprisingly all lost weight (Hashim and Van Itallie, 1965). If, on the other hand, people are provided with as much palatable food as they can eat, they soon gain weight (Porikos *et al.*, 1982).

Variety

An important aspect of what makes food palatable is its variety. People on a uniform daily intake either because they are subjects in an experiment on energy balance or because they are on a strict reducing diet may lose weight at least in part because of the sheer monotony of eating the same thing every day.

Variety has an effect even at the neurological level, which belies the idea that satiety is an all-or-nothing physiological state. Edmund Rolls and his colleagues (1982) have described an experiment in which they were recording from a single neuron in the monkey. The response of the neuron to the sight of a sucrose solution diminished over several trials together with the monkey's willingness to accept the solution. At the end of this time, however, the neuron responded strongly to the sight of a peanut and the monkey accepted the nut and continued to eat several more!

This story is reminiscent of our own behaviour at dinner parties, when at the end of the main course we both feel and claim that we have eaten enough; but some of us will go on to consume a dessert course or even to sample several different sweets! Something like this phenomenon has been investigated in a series of experiments by Barbara Rolls and her colleagues. Using a questionnaire measure of how pleasant food tastes, they gave people foods under various conditions: these involved offering only one food; or a variety of foods in succession. Foods already eaten became less pleasant to taste whereas other foods were rated as more pleasant, and were also more readily eaten. For example, student nurses were offered sandwiches for their lunch, on one occasion with only one filling and on another occasion with four different fillings. The nurses ate one third more sandwiches when offered the four different fillings than when offered only one filling. Moreover there was no relationship between how 'hungry' they said they were before the meal and how much they actually ate (Rolls *et al.*, 1981).

Similar results were obtained when subjects were offered three flavours of yoghurt but the effect is greater the more different the foods are. In other words, if three yoghurts similar in colour and texture but different in taste are offered, the variety has a less powerful effect on consumption than if yoghurt differing in all three sensory aspects is offered. Because appetite diminishes after a food which produces one kind of sensory input (sight, smell, texture) but still remains for foods which produce a different type of sensory input, this phenomenon has been called 'sensory specific satiety'. The effect is not completely specific, as eating meat for example reduces the pleasantness of other meats as well and may elevate the pleasantness of sweet foods (Rolls *et al.*, 1982).

The effect cannot be readily explained by the consequences of absorption rather than the foods' sensory characteristics, as the changes in ratings of pleasantness occur before the person has had time to absorb the food; and nor can it be explained by mere habituation to the stimuli, as the perceived intensity of the food stimuli does not appear to change, only the pleasantness.

It is possible that our preference for variety in food helps us to choose the different nutrients we need for health. At the same time, however, it is clear that variety if it enhances eating could well result in overeating, to the point of obesity. Evidence that presenting rats with a variety of palatable foods led them to become obese has given rise to the term 'dietary obesity' (Selafani and Springer, 1976). Whether this finding was a result of the food being particularly good, or just less monotonous and more varied than standard laboratory chow was not clear. Rolls and her colleagues, pursuing the variety hypothesis, found that rats offered palatable foods compared to standard chow over seven weeks were hyperphagic; and that those rats given a variety of foods simultaneously ate more and became significantly heavier than those given a variety of foods in succession (Rolls *et al.*, 1983).

It is always questionable to extend the results of animal experiments to make assumptions about humans, but this finding does give some support to an earlier one in which people presented simultaneously with sausage rolls, egg rolls, and pizzas, ate more than when served with any of the foods alone (Pliner *et al.*, 1980). If it is indeed true that we eat more in a multi-choice, 'buffet' situation, then it may also be true that with consistent variety on the family table or in our restaurants and supermarkets, we are all of us frequently eating more than we need.

The type of food we eat

The idea that our capacity to eat is limited as is the fuel capacity of a motor car is clearly belied by the results of experiments on variety and palatability. If something is good, or if there is something new to taste, we may wish to continue eating. A factor which may contribute to or in part determine these effects, is the nature of the food itself. This idea is suggested by the results of an experiment in which students were asked to choose some preferred and some non-preferred foods from a checklist (Blundell and Hill, 1985). They were given lunches consisting of either their highly preferred or their less preferred foods (chosen from sandwich fillings, spreads, biscuits and breads) and were asked to rate their desire to eat, their hunger, and how much they intended to eat before, during and after eating. There was no relationship between preference and the feeling of fullness, but two hours after the meal the students' desire to eat returned more quickly after meals in which they had eaten their preferred food, than after meals in which they had eaten non-preferred food.

It has been suggested that the desire to eat may be contingent on the nutritional value of food previously eaten. One possibility is that food of a certain type has a 'priming' effect: for example a hungry person may experience greater hunger after eating a small piece of chocolate (Hodgson and Greene, 1980). It has also been suggested that appetite and hunger may be functions of dietary carbohydrate, especially sugar (Geiselman and Novin, 1982). The theory is that the sight, smell, taste, and ingestion of carbohydrate, especially sugar, leads to high levels of blood insulin; this in turn leads to low levels of blood sugar, which leads to increased hunger and appetite and therefore eating. It is suggested moreover that in eating more under these circumstances people choose to take more carbohydrates in particular as opposed to food in general. Different carbohydrates may also have different effects on hunger. Geiselman and Novin suggest that sugar has a more powerful effect than starch, and Rodin and Spitzer (1983) have shown that differences in intake can result from ingestion of different types of sugar. They gave normal weight subjects equicaloric preloads of glucose, fructose or glucose flavoured with aspartame to disguise the taste. Just over two hours later they gave their subjects a buffet meal. Those who had had the glucose preloads ate on average 478 calories more than subjects who had had the fructose preload.

There is even some evidence that the way in which nutrients are combined has an effect on preference for certain foods. We seldom taste 'sweetness' in isolation but we do enjoy sweetened foods. It has been suggested that a variety of tastes and textures may be important in the development of our preference for certain foods, and Drenowski and Greenwood have in fact shown that whereas a 'fatty' or a 'creamy' taste is on its own fairly unpalatable, cream becomes increasingly acceptable as its sugar content is increased (Drenowski and Greenwood, 1983). Findings such as this clearly have implications in relation to our increasing consumption of high fat, high sugar items such as chocolate and ice-cream.

Some of the results of experiments designed to investigate what motivates us to eat and under what circumstances suggest that to a large extent factors which determine what we eat and how much are outside our direct awareness, and hence in part, beyond our control. This is particularly interesting in view of developments in food technology and the increase in 'hidden' ingredients in our food. Sugar, for example, appears indirectly in many foods (Mintz, 1982), for not only is it used to preserve foods such as jams, and sweets, but it is also used in a more sinister way to preserve or stabilise even where taste is irrelevant: for example in bread, baking compounds, in artificial powdered cream substitutes and in many ready-cooked frozen meals available in the supermarket. It is against this aspect of the food industry and the insidious way in which our appetites are being shaped without our knowledge, that preferences for wholefood with its limited use of preservatives, and for clear labelling of ingredients, represent valuable attempts to redress the balance.

Determinants of taste preference and food choice

People the world over eat a wide variety of foods and flavour them in a number of different ways. There is some question as to how our preferences are established, and how far they are in fact genetically based. In relation to our taste for sweet, our behaviour suggests that we may be more or less programmed to like sweet things. In countries with high per capita income and high sugar availability for example, people consume large quantities of sugar. Japan is a country not famed traditionally for its confectionery but since recent economic growth it has become a sweet-eating nation (Beidler, 1982).

Human infants prefer sweet solutions immediately after birth, as evidenced by their positive and negative facial expressions in response to sweet and bitter respectively (Rozin and Fallon, 1981). Nevertheless, what happens after birth is clearly more complex, and it makes sense that the amount of information necessary to tell us what to eat is too large to be prespecified genetically (Rozin, 1976).

One fairly obvious explanation of food preference is that we come to like that with which we are most familiar. In other words, mother's cooking always tastes best simply because it is what we are most used to. Some evidence for this idea comes from an experiment in which two-year-old children were introduced, each in varying amounts, to several unfamiliar fruits and cheeses. Thirteen out of fourteen of the children subsequently chose to eat the items they had been given the most often (Birch and Marlin, 1982). Similarly in another taste experiment, undergraduates were asked to rate three unfamiliar tropical fruit juices for sweet/bitter (Pliner, 1982). The juices were tasted different numbers of times within the experiment by different subjects, and the outcome was that ratings of liking increased the more often a juice had been tasted previously.

As well as liking that with which we are most familiar, we may also perceive tastes differently according to how familiar we are with them or according to the context.

A preference which is initially genetically determined may be fine tuned as a result of experience. Thus, newborn babies appear to prefer sweet solutions, but the way in which this preference is expressed may be modified. Beauchamp and Moran (1982) tested the preference for sterile water versus a sucrose solution in 140 babies just after birth and again at six months. When the babies were six months old, they also obtained a seven-day diet record from their mothers. According to the six-month records, nearly one third of the babies were used to being fed sweetened water, although their diets did not differ in other respects. These babies took the same amount of sweetened water relative to sterile water in the six-month taste test as they had done at birth, and more sweetened water than did the babies not given sweetened water by their mothers. On the other hand, the babies not accustomed to sweetened water took less sucrose solution relative to water in the taste test than they had at birth. In a later experiment, the authors repeated the test using sucrose in a fruit drink instead of in water. This time there was no difference between the groups of infants, and the authors draw the conclusion that rather than learning to like sweet tastes *per se*, children and infants learn in what foods sweet substances are appropriate. In other words experiences with food tell us in what foods sugar is appropriate and in what foods it is not (Kare and Beauchamp, 1985).

What to one person may be perceived as sweet may to another be perceived as either bitter or too sweet. The way in which people from temperate climates, for example, perceive the taste of fruit differs from the way in which people from tropical climes perceive it. Some years ago, before mangoes appeared so frequently in supermarkets throughout Britain, a panel of British assessors rated mangoes and mango products as more sweet and less firm than did non-Europeans used to eating mangoes, being themselves accustomed to firmer, more acid fruits (Baldry, 1981).

Thus it is likely that not only do we come to like that with which we are most familiar, but that our preferences for and perceptions of a variety of tastes and textures may be strongly influenced by availability and what is culturally acceptable.

While a major means of learning about the acceptability of food is through taste alone, it has also been suggested that we learn about it, or rather are conditioned, through the association of the appearance and taste of the food with the short-term physiological consequences of eating it. Booth (1982) has concluded that appetite for or satisfaction with a particular food results from learning about its value through eating it on several occasions. Moreover, a previously unfamiliar food can become associated with foods eaten with it. Thus a particular dessert, for example, can be attributed satisfying characteristics if eaten frequently enough after a particular meal that has satiety value when eaten in a particular state of hunger. The nutrient that is said to produce these conditioning after effects is starch. The same effects have not been demonstrated for protein or for dietary fat, and Booth suggests that the reason may be to do with the more delayed satiating properties of protein and fat in comparison with carbohydrates.

Having learnt in this way that a food is satisfying we perceive it as good, and may tend to choose it under certain circumstances. Our expectations about how satisfying it is might begin to determine how much we eat and might even override what is appropriate on that occasion. Clearly if it is true that carbohydrate has a more powerful effect in this way than proteins and fats then the scales are tipped against anyone wishing to reduce their weight!

Individual choice of foods can also be strongly influenced by social effects. It is difficult to see how a purely social situation can influence preference for a particular taste or for a specific food, but some work with children does appear to suggest that there is a case for taking such ideas seriously. Quite often food rewards are used to tempt children into doing things they are unwilling to do, and promises of chocolate bars contingent on good behaviour are not uncommonly heard in the aisles of the local supermarket. Less familiar, however, is the idea that rewarding a child with a particular food encourages liking for that food. This has been suggested by Leanne Birch and her colleagues (Birch *et al*., 1980). They assessed the preferences of sixty-four three- to five-year-old children for a set of snack

23

foods, and chose a neutral food, neither preferred nor disliked, for each child. Half the snack foods were sweet, and half were non-sweet. They found that if the foods were presented either as rewards in a play situation, or together with adult attention, preferences for these foods increased. If, on the other hand, the foods were presented in a non-social context or just at normal snack times then there were no changes in preference. The increased preferences associated with using the foods as reward were maintained for at least six weeks after the presentations and moreover they can generalise to other foods perceived by the child as similar to the presented food (Birch, 1981). These findings raise the interesting hypothesis that parents who complain about their children's excessive liking for sweet things may in fact be reinforcing the liking by offering chocolate and sweets as rewards!

Another common practice of parents is to use food, usually nutritious, and not particularly preferred by the child, as a means for their children to obtain some reward: for example, 'eat up your vegetables and you can have some pudding'. In a series of experiments to investigate the effects of what they call 'instrumental consumption' on food preferences, Birch and her colleagues presented pre-school children with milk shakes to which they were neutral, because the taste was fairly novel. In the experimental groups the children had to drink at least some of the milk shake in order to get a reward, either verbal praise, or a ticket to a short film. The control groups got the same amount of milk shake, and saw the film, with no reward implied. All the children enjoyed their 'special snack' sessions, but the children who had to drink their milk shake in order to get a reward showed decreased preference for it compared to the control groups who showed a slight but non-significant increase in their preference for the milk shake (Birch et al., 1984).

Possibly then, the command to 'eat up your vegetables' in this way may result in even less liking for these foods than previously.

The question arises as to whether all foods, other than carbohydrate or snack foods, are open to social influence in these ways. We assume that one of the determinants of what we all consume is the motivation to eat what is 'good' for us and not to eat what is 'bad' for us in terms of the promotion of health and fitness. The power of such considerations does, however, remain in question as evidenced worldwide by the increasing call for health education in an attempt to prevent obesity and ill-health. Some work in relation to the role of TV commercials suggests that as far as advertising at least is concerned, children are influenced in the direction of choosing more low-nutrition foods high in fats, sugar, and carbohydrates; but the same kind of advertising appears to have little effect on preferences for or amounts eaten of high nutrition foods such as fruits and vegetables (Jeffrey, McLellarn and Fox, 1982; Peterson *et al.*, 1984).

It is evident that beyond the notions of eating when hungry and stopping when full, there are many subtle and indeed 'hidden' factors influencing what we choose to eat: physiological, psychological and not least social.

Part II

Pathology of eating

Introduction

Discussion of the cultural determinants of eating and of the control of eating by individuals demonstrates that there is no clear consensus about what constitutes normal eating behaviour.

The problems of definition are underlined further by an attempt to describe abnormalities of eating behaviour and to explain their causes.

The first problem is in defining what are the extremes of 'overeating' and 'undereating'. There is no universally accepted measure of how much any one person should eat at a particular point in time. Therefore the words 'overeat' and 'undereat' have meanings that are purely subjective, being different things to different people at different times. What to one person may constitute a large meal is to another merely a 'snack'. The dilemma is highlighted today by the new publicity given to the eating 'binge'.

The prevalence of severe binge-eating has been estimated at between 2 and 20 per cent of women up to the age of forty, but there is often a discrepancy between what people say about themselves in response to questionnaires and how they actually behave. Given the definition of a binge as 'rapid consumption of large amounts of food within a discrete time period', many women in one study described a binge as having dinner in a fast-food restaurant or sharing a late-night pizza with a friend (Carter and Moss, 1984). In other words it is apparent that a number of people who could be considered to eat normally are identifying themselves as overeaters.

A second problem with the definition of what is abnormal is that overeating and undereating are frequently judged in the context of weight. Many people would be surprised to learn that about 50 per cent of anorexia nervosa sufferers have periods when they overeat – when they binge on large quantities of food only to dispose of it later. Obese people on the other hand may be seen as overeating by virtue of the fact that they weigh too much. Yet there are times, when adhering to a strict diet, that they could be said to undereat; and there are many normal weight people who have periods of overeating alternating with periods of starvation. These considerations raise the question of whether undereating necessarily implies weight loss or whether overeating necessarily implies weight gain.

Another consideration to be taken into account is that under-eating and overeating are in part defined by our perception of the person doing the eating. Ballet dancers, models, and to a lesser extent air hostesses are all expected to be slim, if not emaciated. If they have to eat a little less than other people do in order to stay that way then that may be considered just part of a normal state of affairs. Yet it has come to light recently that a larger proportion of women for whom a slim figure is an essential part of their trade than of women in the general population have abnormal attitudes to eating, and a small proportion of these could be diagnosed as having anorexia nervosa (Garner and Garfinkel, 1980; Button and Whitehouse, 1981).

For the purposes of discussion here, undereating may be defined as eating behaviour which results in a loss of weight to or maintenance of weight at a level which is below matched population mean weight. Overeating may be defined as eating behaviour which results in weight gain above matched popula-tion mean weight or in repeated episodes of physical discomfort and dysphoria.

The causes of undereating and overeating lie on a continuum from those clearly relating to systemic disease to those where aetiology is less clear and where increasingly interpersonal, social factors and intrapersonal psychological factors come into play. Thus in relation to cancer, for example, undereating may be a direct result of the disease process itself, particularly where cancers of the alimentary tract are concerned. Nevertheless, psychological aspects may be of importance in relation to anxiety about the disease or the appeal of available hospital fare. At the other end of the spectrum depressed people undereat for apparently psychological reasons and anorexia nervosa is treated as a psychiatric disorder, although even here the causes are likely to be 'multidetermined' (Garfinkel and Garner, 1983). Where overeating also is concerned there are at one end of the spectrum disorders in which overeating is seen as having a largely physiological basis. For example, certain patients with Parkinson's disease when first seen were reported to show an abnormal increase in appetite which subsequently decreased with clinical improvement during treatment (Rosenberg *et al.*, 1977). Overeating may occur concomitantly with lesions of the hypothalamus or in patients with Prader-Willi syndrome with enough regularity to suggest that psychological factors if they exist must be of minimal importance.

Conversely, overeating may appear to have a largely psychological basis, as in the overeating of people in response to stress.

However, even in cases where the basis of an eating disorder appears to be largely psychological in origin, there are many shades of grey involved and it is often likely that other factors play an important part in its maintenance and in the way the sufferer both feels and behaves. This conclusion is drawn in part from evidence about people forced to undergo starvation in different contexts. A particularly important and often cited series of studies relating to the effects of starvation was reported by Keys and his colleagues just after the Second World War (Keys *et al.*, 1950). They subjected a group of thirty-four male conscientious objectors to twelve weeks of semi-starvation followed by twelve weeks of rehabilitation. As the starvation increased, the subjects took longer and longer to eat meals that they previously would have consumed 'in a matter of minutes'. Food became the main topic of conversation, reading and daydreams; and all other normal activities became restricted. In addition the men bought unnecessary items during the period of starvation, such as books, second-hand clothes, 'knick knacks', and often could not explain why they had bought them. Their scores on the Minnesota Multiphasic Personality Inventory (MMPI) moved from normal in an earlier control phase towards the 'neurotic' end of the profile, and became comparable with the scores of patients with a psychiatric diagnosis. At the same time the men also became less sociable. Perhaps even more interesting is the finding that some months after rehabilitation, ten out of fifteen men reporting back had put themselves on a reducing diet. Hence people who had previously had a normal interest in food and weight had, through the experience of starvation, become concerned about dieting.

All these are characteristics that have been described particularly in patients with anorexia nervosa. In relation to anorexics the reduction of normal activities and in sociability, and the special interest in things to do with food and eating, have traditionally been seen as symptoms of the disorder. The personality difficulties are often considered to be risk factors but in the case of the conscientious objectors they were in part reversed with return to a normal diet.

The descriptions of otherwise normal people undergoing starvation have given rise to the view that a part at least of the behaviour observed in people starving themselves for apparently psychological reasons is due to the effects of the starvation itself. The question that arises is where to draw the line between cause and effect.

The same dilemma is raised in relation to the phenomenon of overeating. After twelve weeks of semi-starvation the men in the Minnesota study were allowed to eat as they liked. In the thirteenth week, many men ate almost continuously. Some developed a predilection for sweets or dairy products which lasted for some weeks. The tendency to binge eat has been described also in people who have undergone enforced starvation as in concentration camps. Murray (1947), in a study of people released from concentration camps after the Second World War, noted that even when food was made freely available people continued to have voracious appetites, to steal food and continue to eat even when too full to do so. Compulsive eating then occurs clearly as a result of enforced starvation. The question in relation to anorexia nervosa and bulimia as they are expressed today is which comes first. The question has already been raised in relation to female dancers and other women for whom it is important to keep up a slim appearance. Now it is being raised also in relation to athletes, both male and female, and runners in particular. Many people are now pointing to an analogy between long-distance running and anorexia nervosa (Smith, 1980; Yates et al., 1983; Leon, 1984). It is argued that 'the degree of body wasting experienced by these starving young athletes is often so severe as to satisfy the major diagnostic criteria of primary anorexia nervosa' (Smith, 1980); and that their behaviour may be indistinguishable from that of an eating disordered person who is engaging in athletics in order to achieve and maintain an excessively low body weight (Leon, 1984). Some runners describe themselves similarly to anorexic women in terms of their family background, and personality characteristics such as high self-expectations and a tendency to depression, and may demonstrate bizarre preoccupations with food (Yates *et al.*, 1983). In some of these people the apparent disorder is, however, fairly easily reversed (Smith, 1980). These people may be anorexics in disguise, but on the other hand they do not as a group exhibit abnormal fear of fat (Goldfarb and Plante, 1984). The enforced and necessary starvation may for some people be itself a trigger for disorders of eating.

There is a close relationship, then, between the physical and psychological effects of starvation and between the factors which both trigger and maintain overeating and undereating. Starvation is for some people addictive, while for others it leads to binge-eating. The question arises as to what are the risk factors which determine the way in which a person will respond to the demands of competition for the beauty and fitness stakes in particular, and to life-stress in general.

4   Anorexia and disorders of eating as a secondary factor

Anorexia or lack of appetite is a symptom most people suffer at one time or another as a result of stress and worry or as a symptom of a short-lived illness. It is a phenomenon that may carry significance at any stage in the developmental sequence, from babyhood to old age.

Psychological causes of anorexia

Food negativism is a fairly common problem in two- to four-year-olds (Pinkerton, 1983). Children who refuse to eat appear to be defying their parents with one of the only means at hand to them, but what is not clear is whether or not this always leads to undereating. Nevertheless between 10 and 30 per cent of children under five years are described by their parents as faddy or finicky and many parents worry about how much their children eat (Dunn, 1980). The severity of a child's eating disorder is associated with psychiatric stress in the mothers, and poor family relationships (Brandon, 1970, cited by Dunn, 1980). However, determining exact causality in disorders of this type is always difficult, and the question arises in relation to children who fail to grow whether they are receiving adequate food intake. One possibility is that their mothers neglect to feed them; on the other hand, living under conditions of continual emotional stress can result in reduced appetite, and either of the two factors could explain the slowing of growth.

Another phenomenon occurring in infancy and childhood which may lead to undereating and consequent failure to grow is that of rumination. This is a condition characterised by the regurgitation and sometimes reswallowing of previously ingested food. Its onset may be at any time from three weeks to twelve months although in retarded children it may first occur at several years of age (Chatoor *et al.*, 1984). It is sometimes thought to have an organic basis; but the infant sometimes appears to enjoy the activity, which is not associated with nausea or gastrointestinal disorder. A psychodynamic explanation is that the behaviour may come to be used as a means of relieving tension in the context of a poor mother–infant relationship (Chatoor *et al.*, 1984). Treatment then rests on the idea of nurturing the mother–child relationship. The disorder is apparently very rare, but can cause immense distress in the parents of sufferers who may as a consequence become alienated from their infants (American Psychiatric Association, 1980). An alternative explanation to the psychodynamic one is a behavioural one. This point of view suggests that the behaviour is learned as a response to the child's environment. The behaviour may be triggered quite innocently, perhaps by a gastrointestinal upset perhaps. Subsequently it may come to be reinforcing for the child in that it gains attention, or provides relief from negative events. Before long a habit may be formed which becomes difficult to erase and which is further unwittingly reinforced by the behaviour of people close to the child.

Failure to grow has also been described in a group of adolescents between the ages of nine and seventeen (Pugliese *et al.*, 1983). These are patients who presented to a clinic specialising in problems of short stature or delayed puberty and who demonstrated these symptoms as a result of self-imposed restriction of food intake. The authors concluded that the patients were undereating due to a fear of becoming obese. None of the other symptoms usually present in anorexia nervosa, such as distorted body image, were present, and also the phenomenon occurred mainly in young boys as opposed to girls, and was fairly easily reversed in response to nutritional and psychological counselling.

Undereating may be a problem at the opposite end of the life-cycle, in old age. There are several reasons why the elderly may have reduced intake relative to their needs. One cause may be as a corollary to illness. It takes longer for an elderly person than for a younger person to recover appetite after an infectious disease and this can precipitate frank malnutrition in a person whose previous level of nutrition was only marginally adequate (Exton-Smith, 1980). Another cause is clinical depression. Elderly depressed people often cannot be bothered to cook, even to eat food, and this is made worse if there is a confusional state. Many old people suffer from dementia which can have a powerful influence over the amount and type of food they prepare and eat. Eating the right food at appropriate times requires a good memory to remember when to eat, and when to turn the gas off; and an adequate level of cognitive functioning to appreciate the use and whereabouts of containers and food preparation implements, and above all of fresh foods.

People in general eat less as they grow older and level of food intake tends to reflect degree of health and vice-versa (Exton-Smith, 1980). Intake declines with physical disability (Stanton and Exton-Smith, 1970). A partial reason for this may be that people with hemiplegias, arthritis, impaired vision, poor dentition or other physical disabilities have more difficulty in getting and preparing the food (Exton-Smith, 1980). A more important reason, however, is that physical disabilities may cause difficulties with the act of eating itself. Physical problems may pose an even greater handicap to old people's ability to feed themselves than do mental ones (Rogers and Snow, 1982).

All kinds of social factors also play a part in the tendency of old people to undereat. For example in conditions of poverty people may have to choose between buying food or paying bills for heating and lighting. In conditions of loneliness apathy can result in taking snacks low in nutrition rather than cooking proper meals. The level of socialisation, numbers of contacts, clubs and luncheon societies frequented, may also have an influence on the level of nutrition enjoyed by an old person (Weinstein, 1981). Other factors might in combination with physical health play a part in deciding how able the person is to fend for him or herself. For example if the supermarket is far away, this requires fitness to walk and carry, the wherewithal to own and drive a car, or the availability of a friend to act as chauffeur.

Therefore in many cases, undereating occurs not as a purposeful act but as a result of neglect either through lack of appetite or for some secondary reason which has nothing to do with the desire to eat or lack of hunger.

Anorexia and consequent weight loss is also one of the recognised symptoms of depression. It is particularly characteristic of psychotic or endogenous depressives, and occurs in about six sevenths of depressed people (Paykel, 1977).

Anorexia may also occur in people with schizophrenic illnesses. In this case it appears that people do not avoid eating merely because they are not hungry or because they are trying to lose weight, but in some cases because they believe there may be something wrong with the food. In a survey of a large group of hospitalised schizophrenics, two fifths had delusional eating disorders (Lyketsos et al., 1985). Some patients believed, for example, that the food contained disgusting or frightening substances, or animals. In some cases patients may believe that someone is trying to poison them, so that they may avoid food altogether, change plates with other people, fast, or resort to vomiting or the use of laxatives.

Undereating in some contexts may also occur to a lesser extent with obsessional disorders, and even in some otherwise apparently quite ordinary people. Food may be avoided for fear of contaminants it contains or if it is served in anything other than the person's own utensils, at home. Many people avoid eating in restaurants or in other people's homes for this kind of reason, or are very particular about the kinds of foods they will eat in different situations, and it is not always clear where the line between 'faddiness' and frank eating disorder should be drawn.

Anorexia and systemic disease

Anorexia and consequent loss of weight are also caused by all types of fever, chronic inflammatory states like active rheumatoid arthritis, ulcerative colitis and Crohn's disease (Hawkins, 1976). Although anorexia on its own is rarely diagnostic of illness, it may be an early symptom of several other diseases such as Addison's disease or acute hepatitis. Anorexia is also a symptom of congestive heart failure. Anorexia may be a side-effect of many drugs, so that in general people who are physically ill may be at high risk of losing their appetite either through the disease process itself or as a result of the treatment.

There is a high incidence of anorexia in patients with cancer. Marked lack of appetite and wasting occur, particularly in the later stages of the disease. This syndrome is called 'cancer cachexia'. It is most common and most noticeable in patients with cancer in one or more areas of the alimentary tract including the liver and pancreas, and in those in whom the disease has spread to a wide area (Shils, 1979). It is not directly attributable to obvious internal destruction, endocrine disorder or other anatomic lesions. On the contrary, the observations of both clinical and animal research suggest a decline in food intake as the immediate cause (Baillie *et al.*, 1965; Morrison, 1976).

The anorexia occurs at varying stages of the disease and for several possible reasons. It appears earlier in some cancers than in others, for example in cancers of the stomach, pancreas, colon and rectum (Holland *et al.*, 1977). Anorexia may also occur at different stages of the disease due to psychological stress. For example, at the time of initial diagnosis patients may lose five to ten pounds in weight, which has little to do with the disease process itself (Holland *et al.*, 1977). Other secondary factors related to the disease may also result in reduced appetite and disinterest in eating; severe pain is one obvious disincentive to eat. In addition the continuing discomfort and uncertainty attached to a stay in hospital, the unaccustomed nature of eating in a hospital bed and the lack of taste of hospital food can all serve to reduce appetite even further.

The anorexia may also occur as a direct result of the disease process itself, for example when it is due to obstruction of a portion of the gastro-intestinal tract (Shils, 1979). In addition the anticancer treatments may themselves lead to reduction in food intake. Operations in the gastro-intestinal tract or head and neck, for example, can produce difficulties in swallowing or discomfort after eating, so that patients may refuse food even when hungry. Radiotherapy and chemotherapy frequently lead to nausea and anorexia.

Several explanations have been put forward for the anorexia-cachexia syndrome of advanced cancer. There is some evidence that cancer patients have an increased metabolic rate which would multiply the effect of any change in intake (Shils, 1979). However the decline of food intake does occur, whether or not there is an increase in metabolic cost (Morrison, 1978).

One explanation for the decline in food intake is that foods taste different and are therefore avoided. Cancer patients, particularly in the latter stages of the disease, often appear to dislike meat and other proteins. In a study of twenty-four women with cancer, Brewin (1980) found that the women described persistent changes in smells or tastes of substances which mimicked changes which had previously occurred in pregnancy. De Wys (1978) tested the thresholds for taste of sweet and urea in cancer patients, and he concluded that abnormalities in taste are correlated with decreased intake of energy, and that the likelihood of developing them increases with body burden of tumour. In common with Brewin (1980), he found that the abnormalities were reversible in response to removal of the tumour or after successful treatment. How far the dysguesia or taste abnormality is a cause or an effect of the weight loss, however, is not clear, as patients who demonstrated the dysguesia already had a heavy burden of tumour and were already cachexic. Nevertheless it has been suggested that the taste changes and concomitant anorexia that occur may develop as a result of a learned aversion to the specific diet consumed during tumour growth (Bernstein and Sigmundi, 1980). This idea is based on evidence from animal work and also from work with adult cancer patients receiving chemotherapeutic drugs whose preference for an ice-cream flavour consumed before drug treatment was reduced after treatment (Bernstein and Webster, 1980). Such an explanation, however, does not account for the similarities which have been found in taste aversion across different patients.

Another explanation of the anorexia-cachexia of advanced cancer is that patients with the disease are depressed. This would be entirely feasible in view of the frequently fatal consequences of the disease and its coverage in the media as a number one killer. However Plumb and his colleagues (1975) compared cancer patients to depressed patients using the Beck depression inventory (Beck *et al.*, 1961) and showed that while both groups experienced the physical symptoms of loss of appetite, weight loss, fatiguability, etc., only the depressed group scored high on the more psychologically oriented characteristics such as guilt, low self-esteem and suicidal ideas. The authors concluded that the use of the term 'depression' in relation to patients with advanced cancer is inappropriate and they suggest instead the use of the term 'emotional dysphoria of life-threatening illness'.

Thus the causes of anorexia are many and varied. The anorexia which results from a purely physical cause is not always clearly distinguishable from that which is maintained for psychological reasons. The term 'psychological' itself can encompass a variety of phenomena; for example the elderly may not eat for largely social and economic reasons, or alternatively they may be unable to eat as a result of the psychological sequelae of dementia. For the young not to eat may be a form of communication of distress to family and friends, whereas others do not eat because depression has the effect of reducing appetite. In all these instances the dividing line between the normal and the abnormal, or between physical and psychological, is by no means clear.

Anorexia nervosa

5

Anorexia nervosa as a form of serious undereating has captured the popular interest in such a way as to cause some writers to draw a parallel with the nineteenth-century attitude to tuberculosis. It is distressing in the extreme for a family to watch one of its members literally starving, perhaps even to death; yet at the same time the 'slimming disease' has a certain glamour, and there is evidence that some family members and friends at least have a certain respect for the self-control of the anorexic (Branch and Eurmann, 1980).

The syndrome of anorexia nervosa occurs mainly in young women and consists of a refusal to eat resulting in below normal weight and cessation of menstruation for three months or more. It has been characterised as a 'relentless pursuit of thinness' (Bruch, 1974), a 'fear of fatness' (Russell, 1977) and a 'phobia of weight gain' (Crisp *et al.*, 1980). Sufferers begin with conscious voluntary dieting, which subsequently appears to take on a life of its own. Often there is diminished insight into the problem to the extent that body image is altered and the sufferer believes herself to be far larger than she in fact is.

The diagnosis of anorexia nervosa can only be made in the absence of any other serious mental or physical illness. The criteria for diagnosing the disorder vary to some extent between workers (Garfinkel and Garner, 1982). For example Feighner's original criteria required the presence of anorexia, an absence of hunger (Feighner *et al.*, 1972). This in itself is problematic, however, as not all anorexics experience lack of hunger, at least until late into the illness. Generally the criterion of a weight loss of at least 25 per cent of matched population mean weight (MPMW) is required (Munoz, 1984; American Psychiatric Association, 1980). However, weight loss may vary between

41

individuals and many anorexics weigh as little as 65 per cent of MPMW or less.

Russell's criteria have been adopted for clinical purposes by many workers. These criteria demand that the patient's behaviour leads to a marked loss of body weight and malnutrition; an endocrine disorder which manifests itself by cessation of menstruation in women and loss of sexual interest and lack of potency in boys; and a morbid fear of becoming fat (Russell, 1970).

In addition to self-starvation, many anorexics also engage in excessive exercise. Others resort to vomiting and purging as a further means of losing weight. Both Bruch (1974) and Dally and Gomez (1979) have described a progression from strict dieting alone to occasional urges to gorge during which patients may experience eating binges followed by weight gain. This binge-eating or 'bulimia' (literally voracious appetite) occurs in about half of sufferers (Crisp et al., 1980).

Most anorexics present for treatment, often at the instigation of family, between the ages of eighteen and twenty years (Vandereycken and Pierloot, 1983; Tolstrup et al., 1985). The onset of the dieting appears to be one or two years earlier but may, according to Crisp and his colleagues, occur at any time within seven years of menarche (Crisp et al., 1980). In Oxford, England, 40 anorexics aged between twelve and eighteen years were referred for treatment from 1967 to 1979, with 75 per cent of them referred between 1976 and 1979 (Margo, 1985). However some people are first seen over the age of twenty-five (Garfinkel and Garner, 1982); and whereas some workers have used a maximum age limit of twenty-five years, Crisp and his colleagues (Crisp et al., 1980) have used the criterion of a twelve- to thirty-five-year age limit.

The frequency of males with the disorder in comparison to females appears to be about one to sixteen (Vandereycken and Van den Broucke, 1984). A characteristic feature akin to the amenorrhoea experienced in women is a lack of or decreased interest in sexual activity which, like the amenorrhoea, improves with the re-establishment of a normal eating pattern. In most other respects, males present similarly to females, but it has been suggested on the basis of over one hundred cases described in the literature that the weight loss is more serious for males and usually a diagnosis is made earlier (Vandereycken and Van den Broucke, 1984).

Eating behaviour of patients with anorexia nervosa

All anorexics refuse food, count calories, and take strenuous exercise (Beumont et al., 1976). They may appear 'faddy' about what they eat, may pick at food, or take an excruciatingly long time to eat what to other people is a very small meal. Some 41 per cent of anorexics avoid eating in public, in restaurants, or even with their families, and prefer to eat alone (Crisp et al., 1980). Some take all their meals up to their bedrooms. These behaviours appear as if in part an attempt to avoid eating but it is notable that some of them are also remarkably similar to the behaviours described by Keys and his colleagues in relation to men on starvation diet, and could well in part reflect or be enhanced by the effects of starvation itself (Keys et al., 1950; see also chapter 3). Nevertheless the hyperactivity of anorexics is considered to be a feature which is exhibited fairly early on in the development of the disorder (Kron et al., 1978). Exercise periods may even occur in the night, thus contributing to a reported disruption of sleep patterns (Leon, 1983).

The amount eaten by anorexics has been estimated from between 200 and 300 calories per day (Leon, 1983) to 900 calories per day (Huse and Lucas, 1984). However, it is of course very difficult to observe the eating behaviour of someone who eats so little, particularly as the eating is itself often a very private affair. It is generally assumed that anorexics as a group specifically avoid carbohydrates. However there is evidence that restriction of food intake by dieting anorexics from all walks of life is not always consonant with intake of high protein, high fibre, low calorie food. While the proportion of protein taken is significantly higher than in controls, and the proportion of fats lower, the proportion from carbohydrates is not significantly different from that of other people (Huse and Lucas, 1984). Indeed there is a great deal of variation in the eating habits of anorexics, just as there is in normal weight people. In a group of ninety-six patients studied by Huse and Lucas (1984) over 37 per cent of patients were considered to be eating diets of satisfactory quality consisting of a range of nutrients. This is not surprising in view of the fact that many dieters know as much about dieting and calories as do professionals in the nutrition field. Some anorexics develop a great interest in health foods, and most anorexics who maintain their

43

weight by dieting alone develop a strong interest in carefully preparing food for other people, although they will avoid eating it themselves (Casper *et al.*, 1980). None of Huse and Lucas's dieters who took food of satisfactory quality admitted to fasting, vomiting or binge-eating. There was another group of patients, however, who took food of unsatisfactory quality, and who in addition used binge-eating and purging to control their weight.

Many anorexics give way to binge-eating, about two thirds of these at least once a week. A small proportion of anorexics who consistently diet also use vomiting and purging, and a larger number, at least half of those who binge, also vomit and purge after many of their meals.

It has been suggested that anorexics who binge-eat or who achieve weight loss by vomiting and purging, are different in other ways also from those who lose weight by dieting alone. Beumont and his colleagues (1976) retrospectively divided all their female patients seen over a two-year period into a 'dieter' group and a 'vomiting and purging' group. There were seventeen patients in the former group and fourteen in the latter. They concluded that the dieting was precipitated by different stresses in the two groups, that while few of the 'dieters' had been overweight before onset of dieting, most of the vomiters had. In addition the lowest weight attained by the vomiter group was higher than that in the dieter group, and these girls were also socially more outgoing than the very withdrawn 'dieters'.

Since Beumont and his colleagues' study other workers too have investigated the differences between dieters and vomiters or between dieters and vomiters and bulimics (binge-eaters), also retrospectively. Some have drawn the line between the dieters on the one hand, and those who also binge eat, or binge eat and vomit or purge on the other; while others have sub-divided the groups further according to whether patients binge-eat or whether they binge-eat and vomit and purge as well (Halmi and Falk, 1982; Vandereycken and Pierloot, 1983).

The most consistent findings across studies have been those of features distinguishing the strict dieters from those anorexics who also binge eat or binge eat and purge in some way. For ease of reference, this latter group will be called the 'bulimic' group. The relative numbers of bulimics *vis-à-vis* strict dieters are fairly similar to the numbers in Beumont *et al.*'s (1976) group, with the bulimics usually about 45 per cent of anorexics (Crisp *et al.*, 1980) but sometimes constituting over 50 per cent of the group (Garfinkel and Garner, 1982; Vandereycken and Pierloot, 1983). While Casper and her colleagues in a study of 105 anorexics found that the pre-treatment weights of restricters and bulimics were the same, others in studies of 193 and 32 anorexics respectively have found, like Beumont and his colleagues, that the bulimics' lowest weight was on average significantly higher than that of the restricters, by about seven kilograms (Casper *et al.*, 1980; Garfinkel and Garner, 1982; Yellowlees, 1985). There is no consistent agreement, however, that bulimics were previously more likely to be overweight.

There is a certain amount of agreement that although patients in both groups were considered shy, timid and well-behaved as children, more of the bulimics could be considered 'out-going', they had more heterosexual experience, and more of them were married (Casper *et al.*, 1980; Vandereycken and Pierloot, 1983). This does not, however, reflect better social adjustment, as the bulimics also describe themselves as more depressed and anxious, more guilty about their eating habits, and more aware of difficulties in interpersonal relationships. In addition the bulimic group appears also to have more problems with impulse control, and consistently higher percentages of bulimics report misuse of street drugs, instances of self-mutilation and suicide attempts, and stealing food on impulse. Twenty per cent of Garfinkel and Garner's (1982) bulimic group reported having made suicide attempts, and 12 per cent had stolen. Twice as many of Crisp's series reported stealing but these were interviewed at a later stage and may have been more likely to admit to antisocial behaviour (Crisp *et al.*, 1980).

There is agreement that bulimics are significantly older when they present for treatment than are the restricters, and that they have been ill for longer. Many of the restricters are under seventeen years of age while most of the bulimics are eighteen or over. In one study the average age of bulimics was over twenty-five years whereas that of restricters was just 20.4 years (Yellowlees, 1985). More of the bulimics sought medical help themselves in this study, and the authors suggest that the binge-eating represents a development in the anorexic illness rather than evidence that there are two different groups involved. The bulimia in this study started on average two years after the onset of dieting, and other workers are also agreed that the older the patient and the longer the history of self-starvation the more likely will the anorexic be to undergo some change in her eating behaviour. This might be a spontaneous change (Vandereycken and Pierloot, 1983). Alternatively the change could come about as a result of treatment, and Selvini-Palazzoli has suggested that the use of laxatives and vomiting may be partly iatrogenic – resulting from forced feeding of patients who are not psychologically prepared to start eating again (Selvini-Palazzoli, 1978). An alternative explanation is that anorexics who binge-eat or vomit are an entirely different group from the 'restricters', with different predisposing factors, and different precipitants to the disorder. Bulimic anorexics may in fact have more in common with normal weight or even obese bulimics than with restricting anorexics. Similarities in attitudes to weight, eating, body image, and in personality may be more important than differences in weight, although the mechanisms involved in maintenance of a normal weight or a subnormal weight in people behaving in similar ways are not yet clear (Garner *et al.*, 1985).

Physical effects of anorexia nervosa

Apart from the emaciation itself, and the effects of the hormone disturbances, anorexia has other negative physical effects.

Some of these are the effects of the starvation itself, for example Russell (1970) reports dry skin, excessive growth of dry brittle hair over the nape of the neck, cheeks, forearms and thighs, commonly called 'lanugo hair'; sufferers often have cold hands and feet, and peripheral oedema. Cardiac abnormalities and arrhythmias may occur, due to the effects of starvation and in response to alternate bingeing and vomiting.

Constipation is very common and there is some question as to whether gastric emptying is in fact slower in these patients than in normal people.

The bulimic aspect of the disorder also has adverse physical effects. For example acute gastric dilatation as a result of bingeing may present a danger (Jennings and Klidjian, 1974) and may occur with rapid refeeding. Prolonged vomiting can worsen the effects of electrolyte abnormalities and renal impairments (Garfinkel and Garner, 1982).

It is also becoming increasingly obvious that dental problems may result from vomiting, a complication that occurs also in patients of normal weight who are bulimic (see chapter 8). In one case of long-standing anorexia nervosa a twenty-five-year-old woman was noted to have fractures of three ribs which were thought to be as a result of forced vomiting (McAnarney *et al.*, 1983).

The measurement of eating attitudes in anorexia nervosa

Slade (1973) has developed a 'short anorexic behaviour scale' designed to distinguish anorexic from non-anorexic patients and to measure the severity of their disorder. It contains items relating to 'resistance to eating' such as bargaining over food, picking at food, delaying coming to the table; 'disposing of food', such as vomiting after meals, or concealing food or simply throwing it away; and 'activity', including taking as much physical exercise as possible. The scale is useful as an instrument for inpatient observation.

Garner and Garfinkel (1979) have criticised Slade's scale on the basis of the smallness of their validation sample (twelve patients and twelve controls) and because it covers only three aspects of anorexic behaviour. They have put a large amount of work into developing self-report measures which cover a wider range of behaviours and attitudes. The first of these was the 'Eating Attitudes Test' (Garner and Garfinkel, 1979). This scale is rated on six points and includes items which are grouped on several factors reflecting: food preoccupation, body image for thinness, vomiting and laxative abuse, dieting, slow eating, and perceived social pressure to gain weight.

The authors point out that the scale does not necessarily diagnose anorexia nervosa in non-clinical groups, although it may indicate the experience of abnormal eating patterns (Garner *et al.*, 1982). In a later study the authors also validated a further inventory, the 'Eating Disorders Inventory' (Garner *et al.*, 1983). The aim of this questionnaire is to tap the psychological dimensions of eating disorders, so that questions relating, for example, to 'ineffectiveness', 'perfectionism', interpersonal distrust' and 'maturity fears' are added to the previous categories relating to behavioural characteristics such as dieting.

Body image and perceptual disturbances in anorexia nervosa

Hilde Bruch (1962) suggested that a perceptual disorder and denial of thinness is pathognomonic of anorexia nervosa. This aspect of a distorted body image and denial of thinness has been built into most diagnostic criteria for anorexia nervosa as a key feature. Bruch also considered a correction of body image misperception to be an essential precondition for recovery.

The disturbance in body image may be two-fold. On the one hand it may result in perceived size being larger than actual size, and on the other hand it may be such that perception of size is fairly accurate but there is a belief that one or more parts are larger than they should be or are unattractive; so that overall weight reduction is desired as a way of making the particular feature less conspicuous (Garfinkel and Garner, 1982). Buvat and Buvat-Herbaut (1978) refer to this kind of distortion as a 'dysmorphophobia'. They claim that 37 per cent of a group of anorexic women studied by them had displayed this in the form of an exaggeration of actual physical defect before the onset of the disorder; and that 5 per cent had displayed an unfounded obsession with an imagined physical abnormality.

Since Bruch's description, however, many other workers have concentrated on the empirical examination of the actual extent of body image distortion.

Slade and Russell (1973) devised a visual size estimation apparatus measuring perceived body size directly, consisting of two lights mounted on a horizontal bar. The subject sits in a darkened room, and has to move the lights to indicate estimated widths of different body parts, as well as widths of an inanimate object. They found that fourteen anorexic patients markedly overestimated their body size while normal women were accurate. This finding was not clearly replicated in a later study, however, where it also became clear that many normal weight women also tend to overestimate their size (Button *et al.*, 1977).

Other studies, some using different ways of measuring body image, have confirmed that anorexics vary in their tendency to overestimate their body shape (Hsu, 1982; Touyz *et al.*, 1984), and some even underestimate. Moreover, using a slightly different method of body size estimation, Strober and his colleagues (1979) found that both anorexic patients and age-matched psychiatric inpatient controls overestimated to a similar degree.

Slade and Russell also noted that as anorexics gained weight they became more accurate in their estimation of body size and the degree of overestimation was also predictive of outcome in that the patients who overestimated the most lost most weight after discharge from hospital. This finding appears to hold up at least within groups of anorexics (Button *et al.*, 1977; Casper *et al.*, 1979).

Garfinkel and Garner (1982) have noted that although the degree to which anorexics overestimate varies, they found, using a distorting photograph technique, that the anorexics who overestimated in a marked way had a poorer prognosis and showed more severe psychopathology than did anorexics who demonstrated a lesser degree of overestimation. However they remark on the inadequacy of supportive data from other laboratories and suggest that while measures of body image are fairly reliable, and have some predictive validity, the meaningfulness of the measure in relation to the construct it is intended to reflect is unclear. They appear to favour a more cognitive basis to the body image construct, whereby the behaviour of the anorexic stems from certain assumptions such as 'that weight, shape or thinness can serve as the sole or predominant basis for inferring personal value or worth' (p. 159).

This idea is of interest particularly in relation to studies whose results emphasise the cognitive aspects of size judgments. For example, Russell and his colleagues (1975) found that when anorexics were deceived into believing that they had gained weight, they ate less and vice versa. In a more recent study anorexics were asked to judge their size using a variable video-image. They attained similar mean values to a control group (Touyz *et al.*, 1984) but the ideal body shapes desired by the anorexic subjects were far thinner in relation to their subjective perceptions of themselves than were those of the control subjects. Moreover they judged the size of a model to be significantly slimmer than did the control group. The authors suggest that the misperception as to what constitutes a normal weight is of crucial significance whether or not the anorexic perceives herself as bigger or smaller than she is.

So, whether or not anorexics perceive themselves incorrectly in comparison with people of normal weight, they believe that their weight and size are too big for them personally and that they should be slimmer. These considerations may have crucial implications for treatment.

Epidemiology of anorexia nervosa

Many workers have noted certain key features of the disorder. One of these is the preponderance of women, such that only recently has it been possible to make a study of men with the disorder by gathering together the data of several separate studies (Vandereycken and Van den Broucke, 1984).

Another notable feature is the over-representation of the upper social classes (Bruch, 1974; Morgan and Russell, 1975; Askevold, 1982). There is a view that this factor in itself says something about the nature of the disorder, which affects only people with a particular socioeconomic status and where certain expectations exist in relation to women. This view is exemplified in the words of Selvini-Palazzoli (1978): 'It is quite obvious that the conflict between so many irreconcilable demands on her time, in a world where the male spirit of competition and productivity reigns supreme, exposes the modern woman to a terrible social ordeal.'

The sociocultural influence, if it is indeed contributing to the disorder, is currently beginning to spread beyond social class I and II. Increases in the proportion of cases from social classes III, IV and V since 1976 have been reported in both England and the United States (Garfinkel and Garner, 1982; Margo, 1985). Also, in a large population study across three psychiatric case registers in N.E. Scotland, London and New York in the late 1960s there were no black subjects with anorexia nervosa (Kendell et al., 1973); one case was found in the New York register between 1970 and 1976 (Jones et al., 1980). Since 1980, however, several further cases have been reported at different centres in the United States, and in Britain three patients of West Indian origin, all from working-class families, referred from the same area to their local hospital, have been described between 1981 and 1983 (Thomas and Szmukler, 1985).

The evidence from studies of psychiatric case registers suggests that the incidence of anorexia nervosa, at least that which is detected by psychiatrists, is increasing (Kendell *et al.*, 1973; Jones *et al.*, 1980). A possible reason for this finding is that a greater interest in anorexia nervosa has led to more people presenting for treatment and more doctors making the diagnosis. It is feasible that in the past women presenting with other problems have not been given the appropriate diagnosis; for example Fries (1974) suggested that of thirty women presenting to an obstetric department in Sweden with amenorrhoea, thirteen women displayed 'anorectic behaviour' in that they worried about their weight and diet, and four were diagnosed as suffering from 'true' anorexia nervosa.

Surveys that are more specific than head counts from studies of case registers, however, have also suggested an increase in anorexia nervosa. For example Nylander in a questionnaire study of adolescents in Sweden reported a prevalence of 1 per 150 girls (Nylander, 1971). Crisp and his colleagues carried out a direct investigation in 9 girls' schools (7 private and 2 public) in England. They identified 1 girl in every 200 in the independent schools as having anorexia nervosa, and 1 in 250 of all adolescent girls attending both public and private schools. The prevalence was higher in the girls over sixteen years of age and the authors suggested that they may have found a higher prevalence overall had they studied an older group (Crisp *et al.*, 1976).

Aetiology of anorexia nervosa

Disturbance of hypothalamic function in anorexia nervosa

Because the hypothalamus has a known central role in food intake and satiety, the possibility of hypothalamic involvement has been discussed in relation to anorexia nervosa.

Lesions of the lateral hypothalamus can cause anorexia and weight loss (Kamalian *et al.*, 1975), and there have been several reports of a syndrome similar to anorexia nervosa associated with hypothalamic tumour (Heron and Johnston, 1976; White *et al.*, 1977).

In some patients cessation of menstruation occurs before the time of reported onset of eating problems; and many patients continue to have amenorrhoea long after normal weight is restored. Russell (1977) has suggested that these factors are evidence of a primary hypothalamic disorder.

However anorexics, and indeed people generally, are often poor historians, and Hsu (1983) has summarised evidence suggesting that it is not in fact clear which comes first, the eating disorder or the amenorrhoea. Moreover, many recovered anorexics continue to binge, purge and starve, so that continued amenorrhoea could reflect the effects of the eating behaviour on hypothalamic function rather than vice versa. Indeed Falk and Halmi (1982) have shown that anorectic factors such as negative attitudes to diet and body image and poor psychiatric ratings are more closely correlated with menstrual status than is weight.

Abnormal endocrine function which may reflect a disturbance of hypothalamic function does exist in anorexic patients (Gold et al., 1980). This does not however imply direction of causality. Miles and Wright (1984) have shown that there is a relationship between hormonal events as demonstrated by luteinising hormone response to infusion of Luteinising Hormone Releasing Factor and interpersonal conflict as measured using repertory grids. This supports Russell's view that 'self-perpetuating disturbances play a part in anorexia nervosa', but again does not offer conclusive evidence as to direction of causality.

Anorexia nervosa as a sociocultural disorder

An entirely different view of anorexia nervosa is one which sees the disorder as reflecting sociocultural factors current in our time. The prevalence of anorexia nervosa in the higher social classes and its increase in recent years have given rise to the view that it is a disorder of modern society. As noted in Chapter 1, interest in dieting and in a slim figure, for women in particular, is reaching epidemic proportions.

Nylander (1971), in a survey of 1,241 Swedish school girls aged fourteen and over, found that half thought they were fat and one third had dieted. The concern with weight and dieting experienced by many young women has since been demonstrated in many other studies, particularly with college students.

It is the author's impression that to achieve a slim figure is perceived by many women as the ultimate achievement, as important at least as either job or social success. The wish to be slim on its own cannot of course be the only major precipitant of a dietary disorder, but Garner and Garfinkel (1980) have suggested that the pressure to be slim experienced by people for whom it is professionally essential so to be, combined with expectations of achievement, are definite risk factors. They surveyed a group of 183 professional dance students and a group of 56 modelling students. In both groups the prevalence of dieting concern and anorexia nervosa were greater than in other students. Moreover the dancers in the most competitive settings, with an emphasis on preparation for professional dance, had a higher prevalence of anorexia nervosa than did the other groups. The authors viewed the results as supporting the idea that heightened performance demands may play a role in the disorder. They noted that music students exposed to similar competitive pressures did not score as highly on attitudes to eating as did the dancers, and concluded that a pressure for thinness when combined with a competitive environment may constitute a strong risk factor for anorexia nervosa.

The direction of causality, however, is not altogether clear. A high prevalence of anorexic attitudes was reflected in the questionnaire scores of Beauty Therapy students in a study by Button and Whitehouse (1981) in which 6 per cent of students at a Technical College in England scored in the anorexic range. It may be that there are certain young women who are predisposed to the development of anorexic attitudes and disordered eating patterns by virtue of their particular interests and ambitions. Beauty students are more likely to be interested in body image and appearance than are other students, and in the same way it would be reasonable to expect girls who are interested in dance to have an interest in things delicate and ethereal which may reflect the nature of the girl with a tendency towards anorexia nervosa. Still an interest in dance or a beautiful body cannot in themselves be adequate risk factors for a disorder so disabling as anorexia nervosa. Clearly there are other factors at work, possibly in combination, that determine which women will, and which will not, fall prey to eating disorders. In one study in an English ballet school, seven girls who met the criteria for diagnosis of anorexia nervosa were identified. When re-interviewed one year later, however, all seven were doing well in their studies and six of them had gained weight (Szmukler *et al.*, 1985). The authors remarked on the difficulty of identifying 'cases' in a group where extreme thinness, concern about weight, and even amenorrhoea are very common. Huon and Brown (1984) administered questionnaires to groups of normal and anorexic adolescents, divided into frequent and infrequent weighers. They noted that the only factor which distinguished the patients from the non-patients was a measure of 'self-esteem'. Although the study was not conclusive this suggests that intrapersonal and cognitive factors are of key importance in relation to other factors in the development of anorexia nervosa.

The psychodynamic view

A view which considers the personal psychology of individuals with anorexia nervosa as of prime aetiological importance is the psychodynamic view.

Anorexia nervosa occurs at or around the time of puberty. Because puberty is specifically a time of growth and the development of adult characteristics the disease is often interpreted as representing a fear of adulthood and its responsibilities.

In psychodynamic terms this fear is seen more specifically as relating to sexual conflict. Early interpretations carried the notion that this sexual conflict is internalised and expressed symbolically through eating behaviour. Eating is seen as representing fantasies of oral impregnation and the wish for this may be acted out through compulsive eating. Guilt about it is evidenced by not eating or by vomiting. Having a full belly may symbolise pregnancy while vomiting may symbolise giving birth (Wilson, 1982).

More modern thinking has turned away from the purely symbolic approach, and focusses on the parent-child relationship as evidenced by the work of both Bruch (1974) and Selvini-Palazzoli (1978), two psychodynamically orientated therapists working independently but who developed their ideas at the same time.

According to Hilde Bruch, the non-eating and associated weight loss are late features of a disorder which is secondary to an underlying disturbance of personality. The disturbance is threefold. The first is a disturbance of delusional proportions in body image and body concept, such that the anorexic is identified with her skeleton-like appearance and denies its abnormality. The second is a disturbance in the accuracy of perception or cognitive interpretation of stimuli arising from her body; this may include the inability to recognise hunger but also a failure to recognise other bodily sensations such as changes in temperature, or emotional states such as anxiety. The third feature is a paralysing sense of ineffectiveness – in that anorexics describe thmselves as acting only in response to demands from other people and not doing things as they themselves want to.

According to Bruch, these disturbances arise from a faulty relationship with a mother who consistently misinterpreted her child's signals of hunger, distress or other needs at an early age. The result is that these patients have 'faulty hunger awareness': they simply do not learn to know what they want, in relation either to food or to other needs. The result is a child who is exceptionally quiet and 'good', obedient at home and at school. The parents themselves perceive their children as perfectly normal, and do not recognise that there is a problem until too late.

According to Hilde Bruch, the parents of these patients are comparatively old at their birth. They are usually middle- or upper-class, their children are well cared-for in a material sense, but self-expression is not encouraged. Both Bruch and Selvini-Palazzoli describe the mothers as appearing to submit to the fathers as head of the family but demonstrating either openly or secretly a lack of respect for them. Selvini-Palazzoli goes further to note that the parents of her patients have intense neurotic conflicts and live in a constant state of tension which manifests itself in petty squabbles. Bruch suggests that in this context dieting may be triggered when the patient is confronted with new experiences such as going to a new school or to camp. She is particularly vulnerable to any kind of criticism and the urgent need to lose weight comes to express an underlying fear of not being liked or respected.

Selvini-Palazzoli describes the anorexia nervosa as stemming more directly from a relationship with a mother who is excessively dominant with the result that her daughter acquires no friends and has no companion with whom to enter adolescence.

In this setting the illness represents a struggle against incapacity and an attempt to regain lost power.

There is an alternative view that anorexia nervosa represents a rejection of growing up, of the femininity that comes with puberty. Crisp (1977), for example, has suggested that anorexics are people who are afraid to grow up. Selvini-Palazzoli on the other hand sees anorexia nervosa as the symptomatic expression of a search for security and power where the fear of becoming fat represents fear of further subjugation.

It is of course difficult to ascertain how far one of these hypotheses is correct. It is feasible for any or all of them to appear to fit in with the picture presented by many individual sufferers and their families.

Many of the studies of anorexics and their families support some of the views of the psychodynamically oriented therapists, particularly in relation to ideas about the functioning of families, the disturbance of body image, and self-esteem and factors that appear to trigger the disease. Thus Casper and her colleagues, for example, have suggested that acutely ill anorexic patients in contrast to normal adolescents describe themselves on questionnaire measures as low in self-confidence, insecure in social relationships, and frightened by sexual thoughts (Casper et al., 1981).

Triggers for the disorder appear to vary widely but in many cases some kind of adverse life event is reported in the year preceding onset (Morgan and Russell, 1975). These may include teasing about being overweight, difficulties at school, or physical illness. In Crisp and his colleagues' study (Crisp et al., 1980) the dieting followed a change in environment, for example one or more events in the past two years such as starting college or work in 37 per cent, and teasing by friends or family for being overweight or having the first significant relationship with a boyfriend in similar numbers. Other significant events were illness in a member of the close family, and marriage.

Pathology in the families of anorexics

A purely psychoanalytic formulation has given way to a formulation which concentrates on the interpersonal, family experiences of the anorexic. It has been the clinical impression of many workers that the families of anorexics have a particular way of relating that is specific to these families and that nurtures the development of the disease. Selvini-Palazzoli's formulation in particular demonstrates this kind of thinking and Crisp, for example, describes the development of the disorder in many of his patients as being maintained by the (albeit diverse) pathology of their families and the relationships between their parents (Crisp, 1977).

From the earliest descriptions of anorexia nervosa mention has been made of the influence of family relationships on the development and outcome of the illness, and removal of the patient from her family was considered to be essential (Gull, 1874; Charcot, 1889).

The problem with most of the more recent studies is that they are retrospective, and information about families is culled largely from case notes. Despite this difficulty there are some findings which appear to be fairly standard across studies.

One of these is the high prevalence of families in social classes I and II, noted by several workers (Kalucy et al., 1977; Crisp et al., 1980). Garfinkel and Garner (1982) noted that 59 per cent of their patients were in social classes I and II.

Another factor appears to be the age of parents. Many studies have cited higher than average ages for parents at the time of their children's birth – but as Garfinkel and Garner point out, this is to be expected in parents of the middle classes and it is not clear which is the more important factor. The marriages of parents appear to be fairly stable in terms of numbers of parents divorcing or separating compared to national averages (Garfinkel and Garner, 1982). However many people have noted a fair degree of discord. For example Crisp et al. (1980) note that out of 105 patients surveyed, 45 had parents where marked discord was expressed, 19 had parents who had experienced threatened or actual separation and in 26 there was 'apathy' with regard to the relationship. Similarly Kalucy and his colleagues, looking at another group of patients, suggested on the basis of a sexual history taken from the parent that 40 per cent of parents were dissatisfied with or had 'disturbed' sexual relationships (Kalucy et al., 1977).

Clinically these findings appear to fit in with the view of Bruch, that while on the surface the parents of anorexics appear to have stable, normal relationships, this superficial normality may in fact mask certain disturbances which play a part in maintaining the disorder.

A history of low body weight or previous obesity in family members has also been noted by some workers. Kalucy has included a history of an actual weight problem under the more general heading of 'weight pathology', where he also includes disturbed family eating habits, and concern about weight and dieting, which he has suggested exist in a large percentage of families of anorexics (Kalucy et al., 1977). Contradictory evidence is presented by Halmi and her colleagues (1978) who compared parents of anorexics with age and social class matched controls and found no differences between groups in terms of height and weight. Having a normal weight does not of course preclude the possibility of having an eating disorder. Recent studies have attempted to estimate the life-time prevalence of anorexia nervosa and other eating disorders in the families of anorexics (Gershon et al., 1983; Strober et al., 1985). Strober and his colleagues interviewed all the first-degree and available second-degree relatives of 60 anorexics and 95 controls matched for age and social class. They found that only 6 (6 per cent) of the controls had at least one relative with an eating disorder, similar to the rate experienced by non-psychiatric patients. Twenty-seven per cent (16) of the anorexic patients however had at least one relative who had at some time suffered an eating disorder. Disturbances in relation to weight or dieting therefore may be factors which predispose family members to frank disorder of weight and eating and to anorexia in particular. It is, however, not possible at present to infer a direct causal connection, especially in the light of new awareness that disturbances of diet and over-concern about weight are more common than ever previously considered.

Another aspect of family pathology that has been considered in relation to anorexia nervosa is the degree of psychiatric illness and symptomatology. Crisp and his colleagues in their study of 102 anorexics found a positive history of mental illness as evidenced by the fact that they reported past psychiatric consultations in one or other parent in 24 families. Psychiatric morbidity was 'judged to be present' in another 46 mothers and 30 fathers, although it is not clear on what basis this decision was made as there had been no psychiatric consultation (Crisp et al., 1980). In addition, it was the impression of Kalucy and his colleagues that 'there are a number of families' in whom there exists 'an unusual incidence of phobic avoidance and obsessive compulsive character traits, an unusual vulnerability to seemingly ordinary life events and a tendency to be unusually close, loyal and mutually interdependent' (Kalucy *et al.*, 1977).

Evidence from more empirically based studies is however fairly equivocal. Crisp and his colleagues (1974) administered the Middlesex Hospital Questionnaire, a standardised self-rating inventory of psychoneurotic symptoms and characteristics, to both parents of a group of anorexic patients. The parents scored no higher than did a group of 'normal' parents of similar age and social class. On restoration of their daughters' weight to normal levels, however, the mothers' scores increased particularly on the anxiety and phobic scales, and those of the fathers increased particularly on the depression scale. Garfinkel and his colleagues in a study conducted both in Canada and in Dublin compared the scores of parents of anorexics and a matched control group on individual psychological tests and scales of attitudes to eating and a 'Family Assessment Measure'. The Family Assessment Measure (FAM) comprises subscales measuring for example a family's ability to solve problems, the degree of communication or mutual understanding between members, and the way in which members express their feelings and interest in each other. The parents of the anorexics did not score differently from the other parents on questions relating to dieting and weight control, or other symptoms of anorexia nervosa, and were fairly similar to the normal parents on scales of psychological functioning. Mothers and daughters, however, did have higher scores than the normal group on four subscales of the FAM, including disturbances in type of family communications and the expression of affect. The authors themselves point out that in the first place their patients were fairly chronic by the time they and their families were tested, and that the results may be as much a reflection of their adjustment at the time as of underlying pathology; and also that there is no way of knowing how far the family adjustment scores reflect those of anorexic families specifically as against families where a member has any other chronic illness (Garfinkel *et al.*, 1983).

Affective disorder in anorexic patients and their families

Interest in the families of patients with anorexia nervosa has intensified as more reports have been published describing psychiatric symptomatology in relatives. Cantwell and his colleagues (1977) interviewed the parents of twenty-six patients with anorexia nervosa and concluded that one third could be given a diagnosis of affective disorder in that they met Feighner's criteria for depression. Winokur and his colleagues (1980) suggested that primary affective disorder was more than twice as common in the relatives of anorexics as in the relatives of control subjects. Since that time several other researchers have suggested that affective disorder in the parents of anorexics is relatively common. Hudson *et al*. (1983) investigated the family histories of thirty-four patients with anorexia nervosa and concluded that the prevalence of familial affective disorder was significantly greater than that found in the families of patients with schizophrenia and borderline personality disorder, and similar to that found in the families of patients with bipolar disorder. The onset of the affective disorders preceded that of anorexia nervosa in the subjects and the authors suggest therefore that their finding does not merely represent a result of the disorder. Rivinus and his colleagues included a control group of twenty-three subjects in their family history study of forty anorexic patients. They got their information by interviewing most of the parents. Their results suggested that anorexia nervosa patients had significantly more first-degree relatives with psychiatric disorder than did the control subjects (Rivinus *et al*., 1984). Gershon *et al*. (1984) report similar conclusions, and suggest that major affective disorder is present in the families of all anorexics to a similar degree. On the other hand Strober and his colleagues (1982) have concluded that familial psychiatric morbidity is peculiar to bulimic anorexics more than to the restricter group.

Other evidence for anorexia nervosa being related to affective disorder comes from descriptions of depression and other psychiatric symptoms in the patients themselves. For example, Hendren (1983) suggested as a result of retrospective evaluation of the case histories of eighty-four patients with a DSM III diagnosis of anorexia nervosa that 56 per cent of these met Research Diagnostic Criteria for a major depressive disorder, and 35 per cent for endogenous depression. Herzog (1984) interviewed a group of twenty-seven anorexics and concluded that at least half satisfied criteria for major depressive disorder. Solyom and colleagues (1982), on the other hand, noted that a group of female anorexics rated themselves similarly on symptoms of obsessionality to a matched group of female obsessionals and concluded that about one half of anorexics are in fact suffering from an obsessional neurosis.

The question arises of course as to which comes first, the anorexia nervosa, or the psychiatric symptomatology which in any case is understandable as a result of having the disorder. Eckert and others (1982) administered self-rating scales to a group of anorexics in hospital and also had the anorexics rated independently by the nurses. The patients themselves rated their depression higher than did the nurses and overall the group appeared more depressed than a comparison group of anxious neurotics, although not as depressed as a group of primarily depressed neurotics. The more depressed patients were the more likely they were to show more disturbed body image, eating attitudes and eating patterns with more bulimia and vomiting; the more likely they were to deny illness and to have reached a lower weight. Also, depressive symptoms decreased over treatment time and weight gain was strongly correlated with a decrease in depression. Likewise in an earlier study, the predominant psychiatric symptom experienced by anorexics was that of depression, but the authors concluded that the overall mental state of the patients was distinct from that of depressives (Ben-Tovin et al., 1979). These findings would fit in with the view that while many anorexics whose outcome is poor have persistent psychiatric and social problems, these problems are secondary to the anorectic symptoms of low weight, disturbed body image and menstrual function (Hsu, 1980).

Other evidence which is said to support the view of anorexia nervosa as an affective disorder comes from treatment studies where antidepressant drugs are used successfully to alleviate symptoms of anorexia nervosa (see Chapter 9). However the efficacy of antidepressants in treating anorexia nervosa has not been clearly established (Herzog, 1984a). Moreover anorexia nervosa is a disorder which differs profoundly in its effect on the sufferer and on families from that of depression. Unless treatment by antidepressant means can be shown to be very effective, with good long-term outcome, the analogy remains circular and has implications which are still doubtful.

Anorexia nervosa as a learned behaviour

A view which takes less account of family and social or psychiatric factors is the view that starvation is a learned response which generates pleasure in anorexics. Many workers have observed the pleasure with which some anorexics refrain from eating and describe the feeling of having an empty stomach, even the feeling of hunger itself. This enjoyment is in part related to a sense of control, and in part is described as relating to the physical sensation produced.

Szmukler and Tantam (1984) have suggested that starvation may acquire reinforcement value for the anorexic. They suggest that anorexia nervosa may be a disorder of dependance, where the dependence is on starvation rather than eating, and is akin to the alcoholic's dependence on alcohol. Like alcoholics, anorexics deny that they have a problem, and starving behaviour becomes salient in the individual's life such that a state of tolerance to starvation develops, just as in alcohol addiction the patient becomes increasingly tolerant and dependent on alcohol. Eating is seen as akin to 'withdrawal', where negative feelings such as tension are experienced. In cases of bulimia, the authors suggest that it is the starvation which is out of control, and not the bulimia. They note that one implication of their theory is that starvation may have an effect on the alleviation of stress due to changes in the brain. This would contradict other suggestions that eating may act to relieve stress and the relationship of eating versus non-eating with mood would certainly merit further investigation in order to clarify these relationships.

An alternative behavioural view which takes account of current evidence about the nature of anorexia nervosa and its predisposing factors is that of Slade (1982). He suggests that inadequate attention has been paid to the consequences of the disorder in relation to its antecedents. He suggests that adolescent conflicts deriving from problems in the family of an anorexic combine with interpersonal problems to contribute to a state of 'general dissatisfaction with life and the self'. This 'setting condition' combines with that of 'perfectionistic tendencies' (Halmi *et al.*, 1977) to generate a need to control completely some aspect of her life. Self or bodily control is the perfect candidate for this as it is independent of the behaviour of other people. In this setting, initial dieting behaviour is triggered by psychosocial stimuli, which would fit in with the view that the disorder has a sociocultural basis. The consequence of dieting behaviour is that on the one hand the individual achieves success or positive reinforcement in the context of perceived failure in other areas of functioning; and on the other hand the behaviour is negatively reinforced by a consequent fear of regaining weight and becoming fat. Garner and Bemis (1982) have suggested that some anorexics may even desire the experience of anxiety and negative cognitions consequent on not losing weight because of the part they play in maintaining the disorder. Similar views have been expressed by Wyrwicka (1984) who has suggested that the behaviour of non-eating, started in order to avoid obesity and hence perceived social failure, becomes in itself reinforced by the feeling of satisfaction about being in control.

Outcome and prognosis of anorexia nervosa

Much of what has been said about the outcome of anorexia nervosa appears to relate less to the effects of treatment than to the course and progress of the disorder itself. Several characteristics of outcome appear to bear a consistent relationship to the nature of the disorder and the way it is experienced by particular sufferers, so that it seems appropriate to include a few words about this aspect here, as well as in the section on treatment.

There is no doubt that some patients with anorexia nervosa, if they do not continue to exist at a level of chronic starvation, may starve even to death. Modern attempts at treatment have reduced the mortality rate from a level of between 5 and 15 per cent (Andersen, 1985); but there still exists a mortality rate of 2 to 6 per cent in several series (Schwartz and Thompson, 1981; Tolstrup *et al.*, 1985). Death may occur from starvation but also from suicide. Bruch (1974) has pointed out that the evidence of intentional suicide confirms the fact that anorexics do not intend, through their refusal to eat, to kill themselves. They do always eat something, however little, and she has

63

suggested that they simply have an overvalued idea of how little their bodies need to live on. Suicide marks the end of the experience of defeat in an impossible struggle with food and weight.

An examination of figures given over several follow-up studies suggests that some 40 to 80 per cent of anorexics achieve normal weight by between two and ten years follow-up time. Occupationally most anorexics appear to make a good adjustment in that despite low weights and remaining problems with eating some 60 per cent at least are in employment (Hsu, 1980; Hawley, 1985).

Nevertheless some 13 to 50 per cent of sufferers continue to be amenorrhoeic (Hsu, 1980). Also most studies comment on the continuing problems with attitudes to eating, food and body weight, and on the fact that on average about half of previous sufferers do not achieve normal eating patterns (Hawley, 1985; Steinhausen and Glanville, 1983).

Certain aspects of the disorder are said to be predictive of relatively poor prognosis, apart from the possible effects of treatment. Patients with very low body weight on admission to hospital appear to fare worse than patients less severely affected. In addition repeated previous admissions for treatment and a longer duration of illness are poor prognostic signs (Steinhausen et al., 1983; Morgan and Russell, 1975; Burns and Crisp, 1984).

Some researchers have suggested that the presence of binge-eating, vomiting and purging are indications of poor outcome; but evidence about this is variable, and in any case if bulimia is a concomitant of a disorder of longer duration then it may simply be a feature of gravity which itself is predictive of poor outcome. There is also some argument as to whether people who develop anorexia nervosa at a younger age recover more quickly than people who develop it in late adolescence or at an older age. Several researchers in studies of between thirty and a hundred anorexics have concluded that children do better than older people and that a later age of onset results in a poor prognosis (Morgan and Russell, 1975; Theander, 1970; Collipp, 1984). However, others have questioned this conclusion on the basis of poor methodology (Swift, 1982); and in a more recent follow-up study in Birmingham, England, Hawley has concluded that children with an age of onset of dieting between seven and thirteen years have an outcome which is in fact very similar to that reported for older people in the literature (Hawley, 1985).

The problem with all these studies, however, is that diagnostic and outcome criteria are inevitably different across studies. Individual approaches to treatment vary considerably from one centre to another and across countries.

Nevertheless the evidence is clear that anorexia nervosa is a disorder which may have extremely disabling consequences particularly in relation to the psychological and emotional functioning of sufferers, and often for several years. It is a disorder which has been attributed many causes, all of which appear to have some validity. It is likely that many factors combine to contribute both to the establishment and to the maintenance of this baffling picture.

6   Overeating and demonstrable pathology

The term 'overeating' means different things to different people. We may all claim to have overeaten after say a particularly good meal or after spending two weeks on holiday in a hotel. Yet the term is purely subjective and whereas one person will claim to have eaten too much on the basis of one evening meal and breakfast every day, another might admit to overeating only after taking a full-board arrangement with additional snacks between meals.

Overeating usually has clinical significance when it is experienced by the sufferer as 'compulsive': when there are bouts of uncontrollable eating with the emphasis being on the lack of control. The eating is, in the words of Rau and Green (1975), 'ego-dystonic'. Until recently however, overeating has aroused most interest only where an observer has been involved; in other words where it is a phenomenon which is experienced as keenly or even more so by another as by the sufferer him/herself. Notable examples are the compulsive overeating of a fat person whose family, made aware of the problem initially by his very size, try all manner of means to prevent him eating; and more particularly the excessive eating of a Prader-Willi child, whose family may be sensitive to the size of every morsel ingested.

The more out of control eating is seen to be, the more likely has the sufferer and also the observer been to impute a physiological or neurological cause. Hence akin to the common lay assumption that people are overweight because of their 'glands' is the more scientific hypothesis of hypothalamic damage, which draws an analogy between overeating in man and the 'hyperphagia' induced in animals by bilateral lesions of the ventromedial nuclei of the hypothalamus. This is directly opposite to the view of the psychoanalysts who might suggest a wholly socio-psychological basis for such extremes of behaviour.

Hypothalamic obesity

Hyperphagia, or uncontrolled overeating leading to weight gain, is linked with the syndrome called hypothalamic obesity. This is said to be present when 'there is an acute gain in weight associated with a defined hypothalamic injury' (Bray and Gallagher, 1975). These are often the result of hypothalamic tumours; but other known causes of hypothalamic obesity are acute leukaemia, benign intracranial hypertension, inflammatory disease of the hypothalamus, and trauma to the head (Bray, 1984). There are several single case studies in the literature describing obesity considered to be the result of hypothalamic lesions. Often hyperphagia is described in these cases. For example Celesia and others (1981) describe the case of a twenty-eight-year-old man who began eating five or six meals a day and felt unable to stop. The cases described are fairly dramatic, as evidenced by the fact that diagnoses are often made at the time of post-mortem; in this case, the hyperphagia was thought to be related to bilateral destruction of the ventromedial hypothalamic area. Usually there are additional symptoms of brain pathology, and this man also experienced progressive weakness of his upper arms. In a later case, a young woman was shown at post-mortem to have a tumour in the right anterior hypothalamus. She was admitted to hospital with hyperphagia and obesity, but in addition had a list of other more disturbing symptoms – episodes of aggressive behaviour, visual hallucinations, reversal of her day-night rhythms – and was too ill even to co-operate for mental status or visual fields testing (Haugh and Markesbery, 1983).

Descriptions such as these attest to the fact that the relationship between eating behaviour and brain pathology is not at all clear, as where pathology is obvious enough to be diagnosed, then so too are many other fairly incapacitating symptoms. In many cases also, there is no evidence that patients with known hypothalamic obesity eat more than other people.

Looking at the problem from a slightly different perspective, Jung and his colleagues (1982) have addressed themselves to the possible relationship between overweight in healthy people and brain pathology. They examined the responses of pituitary hormones and venous catecholamine concentrations to insulin hypoglycaemia in twelve formerly obese women in good health, who had lost weight by dieting. They compared them with a group of ten lean control women who had never been overweight. The results suggested that in half of the obese women, those with familial obesity, there was an altered pattern of pituitary responsiveness and that this may be a result of changes in the hypothalamus. However it was not possible to conclude whether the changes were simply a consequence of obesity itself with a long-delayed return to normal after weight loss, or whether they represent a primary feature of hypothalamic regulation which is linked to a predisposition to weight gain and obesity.

Despite the difficulties of attributing causality, Rau and Green (1975) conclude from the evidence of descriptions in the medical literature of hyperphagic patients with brain pathology that compulsive overeating in general has a neurological aetiology. In support of this they have found, in company with Crisp and his colleagues (1968), that some patients who experience episodes of compulsive eating have abnormal EEGs. They believe that compulsive eaters have a 'primary neurologic disorder similar to epilepsy'; that the cerebral dysrhythmias specifically affect the hypothalamus, or that the primary neurological disorder results in episodic excessive increases in the patients' general drive state. They suggest that the neurological changes could be expressed in different ways in different people, depending on their personality and background. Fourteen out of eighteen such patients treated by them with anticonvulsant medication were cured of their compulsive eating. In a later study, however, only three out of twenty patients with eating binges were found to have abnormal EEGs, which questions the validity of the neurological disorder hypothesis (Wermuth et al., 1977).

The view of a direct and consistent connection between eating and weight disorders and brain pathology is further questioned by the work of Bray and Gallagher (1975). They examined eight patients with known hypothalamic lesions and reviewed the records of a further seventy-five patients in the literature with a probable causal relationship between obesity and hypothalamic tumours. Of their own patients, they concluded that only one was 'hyperphagic' and suggest a role for hyperinsulinaemia with the others. In 2,000 cases of solid tumour they could confirm only 285 obese people, or 12 per cent of the sample. This incidence is no higher than the frequency of obesity in the general population and suggests that the hypothalamic tumour in obesity may be coincidental and not causal in some patients (Bray, 1984). This suggests that the nature of the relationships of the hypothalamus to both eating and weight control are as yet unclear. Only in a few cases can overeating be directly traced to brain pathology.

Prader-Willi syndrome

Hyperphagia is also associated with the syndrome known as 'Prader-Willi', named after the researchers who first described it (Prader, Labhart and Willi, 1956). This is a congenital disorder characterised by hypotonia and failure to thrive in early infancy, varying degrees of mental handicap, short stature, small hands and feet, and hypogonadism arising in one in 20,000 births (Bray, 1981). Excessive overeating leading to obesity is said to appear at around eighteen months to two years (Coplin et al., 1976).

Many of these children are described as having 'insatiable' appetites (Laurance et al., 1981) and a preparedness to eat whatever they can find regardless of quality, such as lumps of butter, or frozen bread. Some children have resorted to stealing food or scavenging from pets' bowls or even from dustbins, and not surprisingly in some cases such behaviour has resulted in inadvertent self-injury (Johnston and Robertson, 1977). Parents of these children find themselves having to keep food under lock and key and some Prader-Willi adults also find themselves under close scrutiny.

Holm and Pipes (1976) have attempted to describe the behaviour more objectively through the use of a questionnaire sent to fourteen families. Stealing food was the most commonly described behaviour; five out of the fourteen families described the consumption of unusual products such as food from the dustbin, rotten apples, sticks of butter, and dog and cat food. Other behaviours described by the families included worrying about food, or about when the next meal was to be, and an obsession with refrigerators and freezers. Some parents hold that sugar intake itself results in a deterioration of their children's behaviour so that they become 'hyperactive' and seek out food even more aggressively than before (Otto *et al.*, 1982).

Caldwell and Taylor (1983) have questioned the view that Prader-Willi individuals will eat anything indiscriminately. They set up an experiment in which Prader-Willi children were encouraged to choose cups of food from a selection of colour-coded cups containing sweet, salty, plain or sour biscuits. They concluded that in comparison with more retarded children, mildly retarded Prader-Willi children have strong consistent preferences for particular foods. This may not prove conclusively that the more severely retarded Prader-Willi individuals have no preferences as of course the test may have been as much a test of ability to colour code as of taste preference; but it does perhaps support the view that at least some Prader-Willi individuals know what they like to eat just as do 'normal' overeaters.

Some other authors have also questioned the assumption of excessive eating as the cause of obesity in these children. They suggest that their energy requirements may be less than those of normal children so that a caloric intake which is within the normal range for their age and height leads to obesity (Holm and Pipes, 1976; Coplin *et al.*, 1976). Researchers who have measured intake directly, however, have shown an abnormally high intake in at least a proportion of patients (Kyriakides *et al.*, 1980) and consumption of up to double that of normal children (Trenchard *et al.*, 1986 in preparation).

As with adults with so-called 'hypothalamic obesity', aetiology is uncertain as there are few reports on brain histology available so that the link between eating and weight and the brain are still largely theoretical. It has been suggested that the hyperphagia results from a hypothalamic dysfunction (Hall and Smith, 1972; Schwartz *et al.*, 1981). There is evidence from endocrine studies for a defect in the hypothalamic-pituitary-gonadal axis (Kauli *et al.*, 1978; McGuffin and Rogol, 1975; Jeffcoate *et al.*, 1980). These endocrine abnormalities may underlie a number of the other clinical symptoms as well as the hyperphagia and obesity.

Kleine-Levin syndrome

Yet another syndrome in which a link between overeating and

brain pathology is assumed is the Kleine-Levin syndrome. Periodic somnolence with hyperphagia were described by Kleine (1925) and subsequently by Levin (1936) and entitled the Kleine-Levin syndrome by MacDonald Critchley (Critchley and Hoffman, 1942). The syndrome has been described in about one hundred single cases to date in the world literature (Waller *et al.*, 1984). It is said to appear mainly in adolescent boys. Onset, which is invariably sudden, may follow a febrile illness, and bouts of excessive sleeping or 'hypersomnolence', or sudden fits of sleeping or 'narcolepsy' may last from three days to three weeks. The sleeping is often accompanied by excessive eating, not in a compulsive sense, but rather of a passive type where the patient eats whatever is available but does not necessarily go in search of food. The type of food eaten might include large quantities of food not normally chosen such as raw meat or stale suet. Terms such as 'megaphagia' or 'polyphagia' are used to describe the nature of the eating in preference to 'compulsive eating' as the food is not actively sought after. Other forms of compulsive behaviour may accompany these symptoms, however, such as fire setting, excessive sexuality, or stealing.

In between bouts of the illness, the patient is said to be perfectly well, and may have little recollection of the 'attack'. Hence some workers regard it as a manifestation of hysteria (Pai, 1950). However, most sufferers are described as being of normal personality before the episodes.

Another hypothesis put forward is that of hypothalamic dysfunction based partly on some single case evidence of hypothalamic lesions on post-mortem (Takram and Cronin, 1976). However, an alternative hypothesis has been put forward by Reynolds and his colleagues (1984). On the basis of sleep measures taken during periods of hypersomnolence and periods of normal behaviour of a patient with Kleine-Levin syndrome, they claim that whereas the pattern during asymptomatic periods resembles that of a normal age-matched sample, the pattern during episodes of hypersomnia resembles that seen in depressed patients. They conclude that the syndrome may therefore be just one more form of depression; in which case these patients may simply come into the category of those who eat more rather than less when they are depressed (see Chapter 7).

7   Overeating and obesity

What is obesity?

Obesity is caused by an excess of adipose tissue, or fat. It is cited often as being one of the commonest disorders of our time and has a powerful influence on morbidity and mortality figures. Hence it has become one of the prime health concerns of the Western world.

Obesity is defined in a number of ways. The most common of these is in relation to the Metropolitan Life Insurance Tables (1960). These tables provide a range of weights for each of three frame sizes: small, medium, and large, for males and females of different heights. Obesity is defined by the tables as a percentage deviation (usually a minimum of 10 to 20 per cent) from 'ideal' weight. The chief problem with this method is that there are no guidelines for determining 'frame size' which was invented by Lewis Dublin, one-time chief actuary of the Metropolitan Life Insurance Company, merely for convenience sake to cope with the wide variation in weights for persons of the same sex and height. One way of dealing with this has been to collapse the three ranges, and to take the range of 'desirable weight' from the lower end of the small frame to the upper end of the large frame, and state that people above this range are obese (Garrow, 1978).

Another common way of classifying overweight is to use the calculation W/H^2 (Kg/m^2) known as Quetelet's index, or the body mass index. For men the range of W/H^2 is twenty to twenty-five, and for women it is nineteen to twenty-four.

Both W/H^2 and relative weight are good indices of fatness, having the lowest correlations of all the weight–height indices with height, the highest correlation with percentage of body weight as fat, and with fat mass. They also have the advantage of having been related to morbidity and mortality data in large epidemiological studies.

Weight-height indices do not, however, distinguish between overweight due to muscle, bone, water or fat, so that someone who is athletic and muscular could be misclassified as obese. An alternative way of measuring fatness is to measure skinfold thickness at various sites (forearm, triceps, subscapular, and suprailiac) using calipers.

Fat people are classified in different studies, often in different ways, using different criteria, as mildly, moderately, massively, grossly, or morbidly, overweight or obese. In general, people of up to 10 per cent overweight are classified as being of 'normal' or 'ideal' weight; between 10 and 30 per cent as being 'overweight' and above 30 per cent as 'obese'. Because of the inconsistency with which other words – mild, minimal, moderate, gross, or morbid – are used, it has been suggested that researchers and clinicians refine the definitions to include categories which are adopted universally (Hanna *et al.*, 1981).

Obesity has been estimated to affect up to one third of the populations of the United States and England (Garrow, 1979). In the United States, the second National Health and Nutrition Examination Survey 1976–80 found that 26 per cent of adults aged 20 to 75 years were overweight, based on a criterion of body mass index 27.8 kg/m^2 or more for men and 27.3 for women (NHANES II). In England in a sample of working people in London 30 per cent of men and 38 per cent of women were estimated to be at least 20 per cent above ideal weight for height (Ashwell and North, 1977). Other more conservative estimates have varied between 13 per cent for males and 14 per cent for females (Office of Population Surveys and Censuses, 1981) and 21 per cent for males and 22 per cent for females (Dawes, 1984). In children and adolescents the prevalence of obesity has been estimated at between 5 per cent and 15 per cent (Craddock, 1978; Peckham *et al.*, 1983).

The prevalence of obesity increases with age, up to about age sixty, whence people become lighter. It affects women more often than men, especially after age forty, and particularly in the 'superobese' category (Hoyenga and Hoyenga, 1982). In Great Britain and the United States, the prevalence of obesity is higher in the lower socioeconomic groups and the relationship is particularly strong *vis-à-vis* women (Silverstone, Gordin and Stunkard, 1969; Stunkard *et al.*, 1972; Hällström and Noppa, 1981). In less affluent societies, on the other hand, affluence is related to obesity in the opposite way, and it is the richer people who tend to be fat (Garb *et al.*, 1975).

The epidemiological aspects of obesity raise questions as to the nature of its aetiology. The existence of both social and gender factors precludes the idea of a purely genetic predisposition and at the same time casts doubt on any explanations which might rely solely on the notion of greed.

Fatness level follows family line, and the probability that a parent or child will be obese is a direct function of the fatness level of the remaining family members (Garn *et al.*, 1981). The fatter the parents, the more likely it is that the children will be fat. Thin parents on the other hand rarely produce fat children. In a four-member nuclear family therefore, the probability of one member being obese is below chance expectancy if the other members are all lean, but around 40 per cent if the others are all obese. The popular view that environment is the crucial factor is supported by evidence that the synchrony in long-term fatness changes of spouse pairs is similar to that observed in genetically related people living together in families (Garn, 1980).

There is, however, mounting evidence in support of a genetic explanation of obesity. Twin studies have suggested that identical twins reared both together and in different backgrounds have fatness levels which are more similar than those of non-identical twins reared in the same home (Brooke *et al.*, 1975) and apart (Shields 1962).

Another way of examining the question of environmental versus genetic influences is the study of the comparative weights of adopted children and natural children and their respective parents. Some studies have demonstrated significant correlations between the weights of natural children and parents in the same household but no significant relationships between the weights of adopted children and parents living together (Bray, 1981). Even more convincing evidence has been described by Stunkard and his colleagues in Denmark. They were able to obtain information about the weights of 540 adult adoptees and of their adoptive parents, and to trace weights of their biological parents (Stunkard *et al.*, 1986). There was a significant relationship between the body mass index of biological parents and the weight class of the adoptees (expressed as thin, median weight, overweight or obese). There was no relationship between adoptee weight class and the body mass index of adoptive parents. The authors themselves admit that such a relationship might not be expressed in times of famine, and that it does not explain recent increases in the prevalence of obesity in the population.

The genetic component is clearly very important. However, obesity is not necessarily inevitable, and some degree of environmental and hence probably behavioural, component exists also. This raises the question of whether under some circumstances people become fat through overeating.

Do fat people overeat?

The arguments for and against the importance of genetic versus environmental factors in obesity have raised again and again the thorny question: do fat people eat more than other people?

For a person to become overweight, calorie intake must at some point have exceeded calorie output. But the question of how this occurs rests on the teasing out of how far fat people are worse than other people at using up or metabolising what they eat and how far they are simply gluttons.

The idea that eating a great deal must alone be the cause of excess calories is clearly not supported by the evidence. We are all familiar with people who because of their apparent ability to consume vast amounts of food without gaining weight have acquired the nickname 'hollow legs'. Between people in the same weight, age and height categories, with similar patterns of activity, there are large individual variations in the amount of food eaten (Widdowson, 1936; Rose and Williams, 1961; Jiang and Hunt, 1983).

The whole issue of whether fat people eat more than others or not is moreover complicated by the idea of a 'dynamic' phase of obesity versus a 'static' phase; that is, there may be a period during which an individual becomes overweight through overeating, followed by a period during which energy balance is maintained at a constant level by eating less than previously. In other words, it takes less calories to remain fat than it did to become fat in the first place (Garrow, 1978a).

Nevertheless, much research time and effort have been

invested in the question of whether obese people eat more than normal weight people. In addition to the question of whether people eat more, researchers have also looked at the question of 'eating style'. Many of the behavioural treatment techniques in particular (see Chapter 10) have been based on the assumption first made by Ferster, Nurnberger and Levitt (1962) that obese people eat differently from normal weight people; they eat faster, take fewer and larger bites, pause less often between mouthfuls and consequently ingest more in a shorter time than do thinner people who are more 'picky'.

Laboratory studies of eating behaviour

One method of investigating the subject has been to observe people eating under controlled laboratory conditions. This involves inviting people either to eat a meal, or to take part in some experiment purportedly nothing to do with eating at all but where food is in fact available in snack form. Food offered to subjects is weighed or counted, or its calorific value esti-mated both before and after presentation; or subjects are observed by means of video-film, or through two-way mirrors. The combined result of most of these studies, often conducted using undergraduate students as subjects, has been inconclu-sive. In an extensive review, Spitzer and Rodin (1981) con-cluded that 'of twenty-nine studies examining the effects of body weight on amount eaten in laboratory studies with decep-tion, only nine reported that overweight subjects ate signifi-cantly more than their lean counterparts.'

The evidence is fairly equivocal also in relation to aspects of eating style measured in the laboratory, such as number of bites and chews and duration of eating. While some studies noted that obese people took more bites, less chews per bite, and spent less time chewing (Gaul *et al.*, 1975), others have concluded that there is no clear difference in relation to weight category (Hill and McCutcheon, 1975; Keane, Geller and Scheirer, 1981; Adams *et al.*, 1978).

Differing eating styles could therefore be characteristic of individuals of all shapes and sizes, and do not necessarily relate to weight category. This was indeed the conclusion of two studies, in which the eating rates of obese, normal weight and thin people were shown to be individually characteristic, and reproducible, even after an interval of one year (Moon, 1979; Witherly *et al.*, 1980).

'Naturalistic' studies of eating behaviour

Criticism of the use of laboratory studies to investigate obese eating styles is based first on the idea that however 'hidden' the purpose of the experiment, obese people are bound to feel self-conscious about eating in this situation; and second on the nature of the type of food made available. For ease of measurement, the food often consists of a single consistency, such as soup or yoghurt, or is in the form of easily counted portions such as snack crackers, sandwich quarters, or bits of cut-up sausage. Thus the food offered under laboratory conditions is frequently unappetising, or has the value only of a snack and is not representative of true meal food.

Consequently, several researchers have invested a great deal of time observing real eating in the 'field', or more specifically in the restaurants, fast-food bars, and campus cafeterias of the United States. The advantage of this situation is that it is possible to watch people eating real, complete meals, ostensibly without the knowledge of being observed. The observers are positioned at the cash desk, where they can see the amount of food bought, or are seated at tables in the restaurant, where they are seen to busy themselves with their papers (on which they are recording their observations) or are positioned near tray-collection points where they can measure the amount of food left on trays after a meal. They are trained to varying degrees in estimating percentage of excess weight, sometimes through prior practice with people whose W/H^2 is known, and to assess by eye calorific values of foods taken. As with the laboratory studies, a number of measures have been used including duration of meal, number of bites and chews, and numbers of pauses between bites.

At least twenty studies have been published on eating in the natural environment since the mid-1970s. In two studies the calorific value or amount of food bought was estimated, at lunchtime in a university cafeteria and in a fast-food shop. Obese women were observed to buy more food than non-obese; and men bought more than women (Dodd *et al.*, 1976; Blackman *et al.*, 1983). On the other hand Meyers, Stunkard and

Coll (1980) who observed 4,412 food choices over six days in a hospital cafeteria, found no differences in choice by weight.

Of course how much food is eaten does not necessarily bear a direct relationship to how much food is put on one's plate, and several people have addressed themselves to the question of whether fat people leave less on their plate at the end of a meal. Some observers have noted that thin people leave as much as three times as much food on their plates as obese people, but the overall difference in the number of ounces is not necessarily significant (Krassner *et al.*, 1979; Stunkard *et al.*, 1980). In relation to style of eating also, conclusions are just as equivocal: the size of bite a person takes appears to vary immensely between individuals and to relate as much to the kind of food being eaten as to the weight of the person doing the eating. Thus, for example, Stunkard and his colleagues gave either a large or a small meal free of charge to obese and non-obese women in a fast-food restaurant and found that the obese women took bigger mouthfuls in the big meal, and smaller mouthfuls in the small meal; and in an earlier study in another fast-food shop fatter people seemed to eat faster than thin but this difference disappeared when people were matched on the type of meal they had bought! (Stunkard *et al.*, 1980; Dodd *et al.*, 1976).

One of the more well established findings of the studies on eating both in the laboratory and in the natural environment is that obese people eat more of food they consider 'palatable' than do normal weight people. It has also been suggested that they are more likely to frequent certain types of restaurant, such as fast-food shops. In one study observers set themselves up in four different kinds of restaurant on one night when there was waitress service, and on another night when people helped themselves 'smorgasbord' style (Stunkard and Mazer, 1978). They concluded that more food was eaten in the smorgasbord than in the waitress service condition, and that there was also a higher percentage of obese clients on these nights.

Obese people do not necessarily have a premium on palatable food, however. In a later study, where visitors to a restaurant were observed at lunchtime, the observers noted that the number of obese people choosing dessert was no greater than the number of non-obese people; and moreover when the positions of the desert at the self-service counter were varied, more people of all weights strove harder to reach the high calorie ones than the low calorie ones! (Meyers *et al.*, 1980). In other words, thin people may be as interested in a bit of what they fancy as are fat people!

However, the question of why obese people should be over-represented at some eating places cannot be ignored. While it is possible that obese people are simply more prone to gluttony than are normal weight people, the rest of the evidence in relation to food choice and style of eating does not support this idea. One important consideration is that what people do in public may be influenced as much by social factors as by any aspect of the food or their level of hunger. For example, in one study observers noted that obese people chose food items of greater calorific value when eating alone than when eating with other people; whereas thinner people chose more food when eating in company (Krantz, 1979). This suggests that while thinner people are happy to make eating a social event by eating more when with their friends, some obese people may be imposing some kind of control when clearly under the gaze of others. This kind of observation casts doubt on the meanings of findings in relation to naturalistic studies of eating behaviour, especially as it is likely that at least some of the people being closely observed in this way must have been aware of the fact despite subterfuges such as dark glasses and disguises in the form of restaurant staff. Even if unaware of the purpose of the observation, many people could be quite discomfited by the awareness of being watched so intensely. This suggestion is supported by the results of yet another study using undergraduate students in which all obese, normal and thin subjects ate more when the experimenter was dressed as a student than when he was dressed as a scientist, in a white coat! (Stalling and Friedman, 1981).

Another aspect of this area of research that may have some bearing on the findings is the possible bias of the observers themselves. In one study the task of observers was to estimate the relative numbers of obese people eating in restaurants providing highly calorific, fancy desserts compared with the numbers eating in 'regular' restaurants. There were marked differences between observers in their definitions of obesity, according to their expectations about what the results of the experiment would be. In fact, however, there were no differences in the proportions of obese and normal weight people eating in the pairs of restaurants (Wooley and Wooley, 1975).

An additional consideration to be taken into account in relation to these studies is the possibility of bias among the restaurant attenders themselves. Many obese people claim to go out rarely, let alone to restaurants where they might be exposed to temptation or, at worst, shame about eating in public; so that there may be a particular class of obese people, with different characteristics from those who stay at home, who disport themselves in fancy restaurants and enjoy eating larger than average portions of delectable food. On the other hand, it is possible that the fatter people are simply hungrier than the thin ones. There is some generality in the finding that whereas normal weight people slow their rate of eating towards the end of a meal, obese people do not (Bellisle and Le Magnen, 1981; Pudel and Oetting, 1977). It may be that some of the obese people seen in public places are more hungry than other people as a result of recent dieting and that this could account for any differences noted.

Yet another alternative explanation of observed differences between obese and lean people takes into account whether the obese people are maintaining a steady weight at the time of being observed, or whether they are in a so-called 'dynamic' phase and are gaining. Kulesza (1982) categorised 100 obese women referred for treatment as 'dynamic' (they had added 10 per cent of their weight in the previous year) or 'static'. She took diet histories over the last four weeks and got a recall of all food eaten over the last twenty-four hours. In comparison with a matched sample of lean women she found that the 'static' obese women had been eating similar amounts; but that the 'dynamic' obese women reported having eaten more. It is important, then, in considering the naturalistic studies to know whether the obese people seen in restaurants are representative only of those who are currently gaining weight or of those who have been dieting and are consequently starving, while those who are currently neither gaining nor trying to lose might be sitting at home.

The question therefore arises as to whether fatter people eat more in the privacy of their own homes than do thinner people. In a study which may have been expected to answer this question, Coates and his colleagues sent observers to a sample of sixty middle-class households with the task of listing the types of foods people kept in their larders and weighing everyone in the family and working out their percentage overweight (Coates *et al.*, 1978). They found no relationship between weight and the quantity and quality of food stored, or frequency of shopping trips; but in any case the subjects reported that 50 per cent of their meals was eaten outside the home! Unfortunately for the study also, none of the people investigated was over 20 per cent overweight.

One other way of sidestepping the problems inherent in observing what people eat is to ask them to record all that they eat over a period of time. The advantage of this is that one has access to a much larger sample of behaviour than in a single meal, but the problems are that writing down what one eats can itself influence eating; people may be inaccurate either because they are not very good at measuring portion sizes or are afraid of appearing greedy, or are simply not very good at remembering, and this varies depending on whether records are made directly after eating or at the end of the day. Nevertheless, self-report studies have failed to show a higher intake of energy in obese subjects either in small samples or in a sample of as many as over 6,000 adults in which dietary recall was cross-checked by interview (Braitman *et al.*, 1985). Spitzer and Rodin (1981) have concluded that more of the variance in aspects of eating behaviour described in such studies is accounted for by individual differences than by degree of overweight *per se*.

Fat people who binge-eat

Notwithstanding the difficulties of assessing whether fat people do or do not eat more than thin people, and in what circumstances, the question is in part rendered irrelevant by the admission by some obese people that they do eat more than others, and certainly eat more than they 'need', sometimes to an excessive degree.

The occurrence of 'binge-eating' or eating large amounts of food beyond the point of feeling subjective hunger, was first described by Stunkard in 1959. He described 'binge-eating' in a small proportion of massively obese patients who came to him for treatment. He considered this syndrome to be of psychological origin and described people as eating very large amounts of food, their eating having an orgiastic quality often in response to emotional stress.

Episodes of binge-eating are usually unpredictable and impulsive, ending only when a point of physical discomfort has been reached. Occasionally the excessive food-intake is followed by self-induced vomiting, but often there is no subsequent attempt to compensate for the extra calories consumed apart from the self-made and seldom kept vow not to do it again. A binge is generally followed by feelings of guilt, remorse, or self-contempt (Wermuth *et al.*, 1977).

Stunkard differentiated binge-eating from what he called the 'night-eating' syndrome. This is characterised by lack of hunger in the morning; food intake around lunchtime may be limited but increases towards evening, and a large meal may be followed by large amounts of food at progressively shorter intervals. People with the syndrome may also suffer from insomnia and may raid the larder several times during the night (Stunkard, 1959).

There has been little real evidence about the prevalence and characteristics of the problem until recently, despite many clinical descriptions. According to Stunkard, binge-eating was reported by three out of forty of his obese patients, that is, less than 5 per cent. This conforms fairly well with the popular view of dieting that has held until recently. Although few obese people who attempt to diet ever achieve their desired weight let alone maintain it, the popular view as represented in the women's press even now is that anyone can successfully control her weight by effecting a simple change in diet (Parham *et al.*, 1986). By implication, binge-eating does not exist or is unimportant. In this atmosphere of denial, it is indeed tempting for the obese person faced perhaps for the first time with a dietician optimistically proffering a 1,000 calorie diet sheet, to refrain from mentioning a binge-eating problem at all.

More recently, however, Hilde Bruch, a psychiatrist who has treated hundreds of individuals with eating problems, reported that almost all of her obese patients have displayed binge-eating at one time or another (Bruch, 1974). Her sample is of course biased by the fact that these are people who have chosen to consult a psychiatrist, but in the author's own experience at least half of patients randomly selected from those attending for the first time at a hospital obesity clinic admitted that they sometimes binged. Many of these people were relieved to relate episodes of overeating which they described as taking on a life of their own. Once embarked on, an eating binge is almost impossible to stop, and afterwards the patient can recall the quantity eaten only with difficulty.

In a survey of 280 grossly overweight participants in a weight-control programme, 28 per cent reported themselves as binge-eating regularly or at least twice a week prior to treatment; and an additional 22 per cent reported frequent binge-eating or at least one episode per week (Loro and Orleans, 1981). The prevalence of binge-eating appears to be similar also in mildly to moderately overweight people (Jackson and Ormiston, 1977). Possibly the contrast with Stunkard's earlier figure can be explained by the use of self-report questionnaires where people are asked about the problem, which in itself implies permission to discuss it, in comparison with a situation where people may or may not divulge information of their own volition.

Binge-eating has been thought to occur more frequently among women than among men. However Loro and Orleans found that approximately 50 per cent of both men and women had engaged in regular or frequent binge-eating, and if there is a difference it may be rather in relation to the nature of the causes or triggers than to the incidence itself (Edelman, 1981).

In order to establish the exact nature of a binge we have of necessity to rely on self-report. By its very nature, a binge is unavailable for direct observation. Binge-eaters do it in private, isolating themselves often secretly, from families and friends prior to and during a binge. This of course makes definition extremely difficult, and as to how much food is consumed, the evidence is necessarily anecdotal. Sufferers report eating varying amounts, and this again depends often on the nature of their relationship with the interviewer. Typical amounts might range from a subjectively large meal, through to double portions of dessert, whole packets of biscuits or pudding mix, to two or three meals eaten one after the other and followed by several bowls of cereal, tinned fruit and ice-cream. Stunkard (1959), from the reports of one of his patients, estimated a possible total of 20,000 calories in an extended binge. Other more conservative reports indicate considerable variation, and

83

the amount consumed on any one occasion may vary from 1,000 to 10,000 calories (Loro and Orleans, 1981; Swanson and Dinello, 1970).

The kind of food preferred is often high in calories, and many people tend to choose 'junk food' such as chocolates, cakes, biscuits, or foods needing little preparation such as packets of cereal, sandwiches, ready-made desserts.

A binge episode may be triggered merely by seeing, tasting or being offered a preferred food; it is almost as though some dieters are 'addicted' to certain foods, being unable to resist them and therefore needing to avoid them at all costs.

Another common explanation given by binge-eaters is that they eat in response to emotional stress – tension, anxiety, loneliness, boredom; or as a result of interpersonal conflict and often annoyance or anger. As a result of the binge-eating, people typically feel physically tired, groggy, bloated, sleepy or sluggish; the concomitant psychological state is frequently one of relief, calm, relaxation, and all uncomfortable thoughts are (albeit temporarily) obliterated. Frequently, however, these thoughts and feelings, if present, are followed by guilt, self-disgust and misery. The pattern may be self-reinforcing in that a vicious cycle of negative thoughts or experiences leading to eating, to numbness and hence to guilt and hence to eating again, is set up, a pattern which in effect is very similar to that seen in other states of psychological dependence or addiction.

Causes of overeating in obese people

Despite the difficulties inherent in assessing whether or not fat people eat more than thin people, still the assumption has often been made that they do, and this has formed the basis of much of the available literature on the causes of overeating.

Perception of taste and satiety

One area that has been widely investigated is the question of how obese people experience hunger and satiety. This is based on the assumption that people will gain weight if there is some fault in the mechanism which tells them when to stop and when to start eating. If there is such a fault in the satiety mechanism then obese people could be expected to respond even less accurately than do thin people to disguised preloads (see Chapter 2).

Some workers have suggested that this is in fact the case; that given a drink, for example, of disguised calorific value, obese people will drink more and take longer to reach satiety than thin people (Linton *et al.*, 1972).

On the whole, however, the evidence from preload studies suggests that obese people are no less accurate than are normal weight people in relation to knowing how many calories they have consumed (Wooley, 1972; Durrant *et al.*, 1982). Obese and normal weight people alike eat more and put on weight when food is plentiful and good (Porikos *et al.*, 1977).

An alternative approach has been to examine taste perception in obese people. The idea behind this area of work is that if obese people taste food differently or are more responsive to sweet taste then they will be likely to eat more than thinner people. It has been suggested that heavy infants consume more sweetened formula in proportion to their weight than do normal weight or low birth-weight infants (Nisbett and Gurwitz, 1970). However, as we have seen in Chapter 2, weight is only one of several variables that may affect preference or intake, and it may be dangerous to draw conclusions of this kind. Indeed other workers have demonstrated that variations in taste responsiveness within weight groups may be greater than that between groups (Witherly *et al.*, 1980) and that there are people in all weight categories who are either highly or marginally responsive to sweet taste (Thompson *et al.*, 1976). Joel Grinker (1978) in a series of studies in her laboratory has also shown that obese people are not more sensitive to sweet taste and that in fact the judgments of adults and children are as much influenced by attributes other than sweetness, such as colour.

Another application of the taste perception approach is based on the idea that the pleasantness of taste and smell of food varies with physiological state. Cabanac and Duclaux (1970) reported that after a glucose preload taken orally or tubed directly to the stomach, people found the taste of a sucrose solution less pleasant than previously. Cabanac and his colleagues went on to report that this reduction in rated pleasantness of a sucrose solution was less marked in obese people than in thin people (Cabanac *et al.*, 1971). In other words, they implied that there is a kind of sensory feedback as a result of ingesting nutrients which controls body weight and which is faulty or absent in obese people. Other studies, however, have reported that obese subjects decrease their taste preferences for sweet stimuli following caloric preloads, just as do normals (Thompson *et al.*, 1976) or that if there is a difference between obese and normal weight people this may be due to greater individual variability in the obese response (Frijters and Rasmüssen-Conrad, 1982). There is some question, however, as to whether high and low calorie preloads produce significant differences in reported pleasantness ratings of sucrose solutions at all (Wooley *et al.*, 1972). Even where differences are noted, it is possible that these may relate to the phenomenon of dieting and deprivation as much as to being fat *per se*. For example 'reduced' obese people show preferences for sweetened high fat foods greater than those of normal weight and obese people (Drenowski *et al.*, 1983).

Hunger and salivation

Yet one more way of looking at the possible differences between obese and normal weight people has been to investigate the 'hunger' end of the process; to ask the question 'do fat people get more hungry or are their bodies telling them they need to eat more often in response to more situations than are those of normal weight people?' As usual where psychological/physiological research is concerned researchers have preferred to find some measurable, automatic response rather than simply asking people outright: do you feel like eating now? They have chosen the salivation response which since the time of Pavlov has been viewed as a conditioned and therefore automatic and not necessarily conscious response to the anticipation of food.

The Wooleys (1973) were the first people to suggest that salivation was a reliable involuntary measure of appetite in human subjects. They measured the amount of saliva collected on dental rolls in the mouth and found that salivation was raised when people were asked to look at or think about palatable food. They subsequently found that obese people salivated more than normal weight people in response to being presented with palatable foods. Yet while there is some support for this finding of a difference in response between obese and normal weight people (Sahakian, 1982), other workers have not found a relationship between degree of overweight and measures of salivation (Nirenberg and Miller, 1982).

The Wooleys also found that while normal weight people salivated more after a low calorie than after a high calorie preload, obese people's responses did not vary in relation to the amount previously eaten. The implication of this is that obese people are less sensitive to the energy changes in the diet, or in other words cannot sense when they have eaten enough. Again the evidence is equivocal. Contradictory results were described by Durrant and Royston (1979) who found that salivation in obese people increased with level of previous deprivation; in other words they suggest that obese people are responsive to differences in energy intake. Some of the contradictions might be explained, however, by differences in procedure, and some by differences between individuals. Salivation varies immensely between individuals and from day to day (Durrant, 1981; Brummer and Pudel, 1981). One explanation for this takes into account the fact that whether fat or thin, people may be experiencing different levels of acute deprivation. Over a three-week period, the level of salivation in obese people fed decreasing numbers of calories was reduced, and increased again with more calories (Durrant, 1981). A similar result was reported by Rosen (1981) whose subjects were dieted under supervision for six weeks; salivary response to pizza decreased over time. Therefore the differences in results between studies may be due less to how obese or not people are than to their level of deprivation, or in other words how long they have been dieting, at the time.

Other studies have found that people on self-imposed diets or who are currently gaining weight actually show increased salivation in response to food presentation (Klajner et al., 1981; Guy-Grand and Goga, 1981). It has been suggested that some obese people and dieters are really 'hungry' because their weight is below 'set-point' and that the increased salivation is a sign of the body's attempt to return to its correct weight. The decreased salivation seen with deprivation in some studies on the other hand may be a sign of inhibitory conditioning having lowered the normal salivary response to palatable food (Herman *et al.*, 1981). In this case the deprived person has learned that food is in short supply and the salivation response is inhibited as with Pavlov's dogs when they learn that food when accompanied by a particular signal will not be forthcoming.

The differences between the ways in which fat people and thin people experience hunger and satiety or respond to the appearance and taste of food may be no greater than the differences that exist between individuals. The extent of the differences that do exist is unclear, and some of them may be explained by the dieting status of individuals. Fat people are often on diets, or think they should be, whereas thin people are less likely to be.

The psychology of obese people

It can be seen from the foregoing discussions that the phenomenon of overweight is traditionally perceived as being synonymous with that of overeating. This being so, attempts to describe the psychopathology of obese people have often carried the implication that they overeat. Descriptions of psychopathology and personality offer explanations for excessive eating as often as they characterise the dilemma of being fat.

Obesity and depression

There is a view that obesity and overeating arise as a 'defence' against depression (Kornhaber, 1970). If this were so, then to stop eating should result in depression, and to go on a diet would, to take an extreme view, lead to psychiatric disorder. As yet there is no evidence that people who stop binge-eating become depressed, but such is the misery of some obese people on diets that many are referred to the psychiatric clinic. Of course people who are miserable because they are overweight or are trying not to be do not necessarily qualify for psychiatric diagnosis, and whether or not a fat person receives psychiatric treatment may depend on the orientation of the psychiatrist concerned.

Nevertheless, some workers in the field of obesity have addressed themselves seriously to the question of whether obese people are more or less depressed or anxious than other people and of whether losing weight on a diet results in more or less depression or anxiety.

Clinical depression is usually said to be associated with decreased appetite. However there are some people, women in particular, who when depressed eat more and gain weight rather than losing weight. This phenomenon accounts for possibly one seventh of depressed people (Paykel, 1977). This has raised the question of whether fat people are necessarily depressed. In a study of eighty patients about to have gastric bypass operations, Katherine Halmi and her colleagues noted that just over 28 per cent of the patients were either suffering from or had at some stage in their lives experienced clinical depression (Halmi *et al.*, 1980). They suggested, however, that this represents a lifetime prevalence no higher than that in the population in general. They did not mention how many of the patients had actually gone for treatment for their depression, and in a later study Hopkinson and Bland argued that this is a critical factor (Hopkinson and Bland, 1982). They themselves studied a group of seventy-three consecutive grossly obese potential candidates for surgical treatment of their obesity, nearly one fifth of whom reported having at least one primary depression requiring treatment, and the authors suggest that this is higher than the expectancy for treated lifetime depression found in the normal population.

There is little agreement, then, about the prevalence of clinical depression among obese people. The conclusion which several researchers make, however, is that many super-obese people suffer from depressive moods with or without the existence of depression which could be diagnosed according to strict criteria. For example nearly 80 per cent of Hopkinson and Bland's (1982) sample reported periodic depressive moods lasting from hours for some people to one week for others. In another study, both patients about the have gastric surgery and normal obese patients described themselves as more depressed than normal weight people on the Zung self-rating scale, but again this did not reach clinical proportions (Bull *et al.*, 1983).

The existence of an association of fatness with depression or depressed moods does not tell us whether it is the depression that caused the overeating, or whether overweight people are depressed because they are fat. Another possibility is that only the most disturbed and hence depressed people seek treatment. It is in fact likely that whereas many obese people undergoing medical or psychiatric treatment show psychiatric disturbance, obese people in the general population show comparable or better functioning than non-obese people (McReynolds, 1982).

Another way of looking at the problem is to suggest that fatness is a 'defence' against the experience of depression. It has been suggested that some groups of fat people, in particular men over the age of forty, and younger middle-class women, are less depressed and anxious than people of normal weight (Crisp et al., 1980a) As a corollary to this it might be expected that on the one hand people would become more depressed as they lost weight, or that on the other hand overeating would be used as a means of warding off depression.

In support of this idea, some people have in fact found that patients on diets report an increase in the experience of depressed moods. Stunkard and Rush (1974) concluded in a review paper that 'there is a high incidence of symptoms of emotional illness in outpatients treated for obesity'. They quoted previous work by Stunkard in which he concluded on the basis of retrospective reports by patients of previous attempts to reduce that emotional symptoms affected 80 per cent of the group. They also quoted another study in which 26 per cent of a group became less depressed and anxious with successful dieting and concluded that the 74 per cent who dropped out must have done so because dieting had the effect of increasing depression (Shipman and Plesset, 1963).

It is possible, however, that depression is associated with unsuccessful dieting rather than weight loss per se. In support of this alternative view, other researchers have noted that depression decreases with weight loss, and that moreover the more weight is lost, the greater the improvement in self-ratings of mood (Wing et al., 1984; Ley, 1984).

So whereas a few people may become fat because they are depressed, others are depressed because they are fat and cannot diet, and still others may not become depressed at all.

Obesity and personality

An alternative explanation for differences between obese and non-obese people has been that they differ in underlying personality.

Fat people in general are no more neurotic than are thin people (Silverstone, 1968). In an outpatient study of patients who were at least 10 kilograms over their maximum weight for height, female patients did describe themselves on the Eysenck Personality Inventory as on average as high in Neuroticism as a group of mixed Neurotics (Gilbert and Garrow, 1983). This finding is not unusual, however, in groups of outpatients with chronic medical problems such as arthritis or irritable bowel syndrome, and begs the question yet again of whether the very overweight people are neurotic because they are fat or fat because they are neurotic.

The same problem arises in relation to other tests of personality also. Several researchers have attempted to differentiate between obese and non-obese people by means of personality questionnaires. The Minnesota Multiphasic Personality Inventory has been frequently used. Some studies have suggested that obese people are differentiated from non-obese people by higher scores on the Depressive and Psychasthenia scales (Held and Snow, 1972; Levitt and Fellner, 1965). In a more recent study obese patients were divided into three groups on the basis of their scores on the MMPI. The first group had no elevated scores which suggested that these people had adequate psychological resources; the second group scored high on depression and social introversion and the third group scored high on scales which in combination suggested that they might have high levels of anger and hostility, directed outwards so that they could be expected to have problems in social relationships (Duckro *et al.*, 1983). Other researchers on the other hand have found no differences between obese and normal weight people on the 'Minimult', a shortened version of the MMPI (Igoin and Apfelbaum, 1982) or on other similar kinds of pencil and paper test (Keith and Vandenberg, 1974).

All of this points emphasis to the idea that while some obese people may have problems with personality or with relationships with other people, or simply with the problems attendant upon above average fatness, others may function perfectly normally in terms of their personal psychology. Just as it is difficult to characterise the eating behaviour of the fat person, so it is nearly impossible to characterise the average fat person as neurotic or depressed, or by any particular dimension of personality. Nevertheless attempts have been made to predict which people might do well on diets in relation to scores on personality tests, the assumption being that at least some obese people have poor control, and that this can be predicted on measures of personality. This aspect will, however, be discussed in a later chapter.

Obesity and body image

Another idea that has received some attention is that of body image. Just as a distorted body image has been regarded in underweight persons as a criterion for the degree of eating disorder, so too has it received some attention in relation to obese people.

Many fat people describe themselves as being immensely unhappy with the way they look, an unhappiness that is accompanied often by low self-esteem in general. In children at least there appears to be some relationship between 'body-esteem' and self-esteem which holds true both for fat and for thin children (Mendelson and White, 1982). The way a person sees himself is bound to have an effect on the way in which he or she behaves, and it might be expected that body image would therefore have a powerful influence over the way in which he or she deals with food. In other words, we might expect the person who feels fat to behave differently in some way from other people, either by eating more, or by acting 'fat' or by eating less in an effort to become thinner. The very intense relationship that a fat person may have with her body, almost as with another person, is painfully expressed in a poem written by a patient battling with her diet time after time:

You surround me. You smother me. You insult me.
Because of you, I am self-conscious – afraid to meet people;
Afraid of their opinion of me.
You turn me into a vast object – able to converse with either sex, because I have no sex.
I hate you. I hate myself for creating you.
You make me tired, exhausted.
I can't see my feet – can't tie my shoe laces – can't bend down.
I feel dowdy and useless a gargantuan vegetable.

You are a parasite, a leech sapping my strength.
People think I am simple because of you.
They mouth their words and talk slowly and loudly at me.
I always end up doing the washing up at parties –
Glad to escape from the food and the trivial conversation –
To the comparative haven of peace of the kitchen.
But now the tables are turning.
I'm slowly murdering you.
I can pinch you.
It is as if I could take my french cook's knife
And slice you to pieces.
You are gradually disappearing from my body and my life.
How I abhor you.
You are my fat.

The response to one's physical characteristics as unattractive or undesirable is commonly experienced by people who are fat, as assessed by questionnaires, line drawings and sentence completion tests.

What is less certain is how far obese people have images of their bodies which are distortions of reality. Various measures of body image have been used, from verbal descriptions to estimations of body dimensions using visual size estimation apparatus, to confrontation with variable video pictures which have to be adjusted to produce the perceived dimensions of the person. The problem with these various measures is that results are neither reliable nor valid and many researchers have produced different results (McCrea et al., 1982).

Some workers have suggested that obese people are fairly accurate at estimating their true size (Schiebel and Castelnuovo-Tedesco, 1977; Speaker et al., 1983). Many others have suggested however that obese people overestimate their width just as do anorexics (Slade and Russell, 1973; Glucksman and Hirsch, 1968; McCrea and Summerfield, 1983). This finding becomes of utility, however, only in so far as it represents a distortion of body image which is in some way predictive of behaviour. Not all obese people behave in the same way in terms of eating habits, or in relation to how much they eat, and in the same way a phenomenon which exists in all obese people alike is unlikely to shed light on the aetiology or maintenance of overweight. It is possible, however, that the findings in relation to body image are true only in groups of people who profess to have a problem. In a related study, Storz (1982) compared obese adolescent girls in high school with obese girls who had sought help in a clinic in Philadelphia. Those girls who were asking for help with weight reduction perceived themselves as significantly heavier than did their counterparts in the classroom. It is feasible that those people who present for treatment are a different group in terms of the way in which they see themselves from those, perhaps equally obese people, who do not.

The Internal-External Hypothesis

One hypothesis to which a great deal of attention has been paid in relation to the establishment and maintenance of overeating and obesity is the Internal-External Hypothesis advanced by Schachter and his colleagues in the late 1960s.

Schachter held that whereas normal weight people eat in response to internal physiological stimuli or hunger, obese people eat primarily in response to immediate external cues associated with food, such as the time of day, the sight and visual prominence of food, and the sight of people eating. For example, in one study Schachter and his colleague altered the clocks so as to trick people into believing it was near to dinner time (Schachter and Gross, cited in Schachter, 1968). The obese subjects in the study ate almost twice as many snack crackers when they believed the time was just after 6 p.m. than when they believed it to be 5.20 p.m. For normal weight people, on the other hand, the trend was in the opposite direction, as if they were saving themselves for their dinners. In another study in which shelled almonds were available, nearly all obese subjects ate them, but when the almonds were unshelled, only one out of nineteen obese people ate them. As further evidence for the theory that obese people respond more to external than to internal cues, Schachter points out that larger numbers of obese than of normal weight Jews observe the fast on the Day of Atonement, his explanation being that as food cues are absent, fasting is easier for the fatter people.

The theory is much cited, and does have a certain common sense appeal. It has contributed to the basis of much of the behavioural treatment of obesity, where emphasis is put on avoidance of eating in response to external cues such as the time of day or the sight of good food

There are, however, many problems with the theory, many of which have been expressed in detail by Rodin, who has herself conducted a great deal of the research in the area. As a result of testing hundreds of subjects of all weights, she and others have found that degree of overweight is not well correlated with degree of responsiveness to external cues (Rodin, 1981). In other words, people of normal weight may be as responsive to external food cues as are obese people. For example, Rodin and Slochower (1976) demonstrated that when girls at a holiday camp were given free access to as much good food as they liked, externally responsive girls of normal weight began to increase their intake and to gain weight. They subsequently began to lose the weight again, which also raises the question of why it is that some externally responsive people become more obese than others, or stay that way once having gained the weight.

Another problem with the theory is the assumption that people of normal weight respond to internal cues like gastric motility. We now know that people of all weights have difficulty in knowing how much they have eaten (see Chapter 2), and that in any case it is not clear how far gastric hunger contractions themselves influence when we start to eat and how much we eat.

Schachter's theory also postulates some explanation for a possible relationship in obese people between eating and anxiety. It is clear from studies of binge-eating that many people see themselves as eating in response to anxiety. While people of normal weight have also admitted to eating in response to anxiety or negative mood states such as boredom it is generally assumed that normal weight people eat less when anxious. Schachter predicts that as obese people do not respond to internal cues, they will, unlike people of normal weight, continue to eat the same amount when made anxious. In other words, because the obese person is not aware of internal hunger and satiety cues, he also does not respond to the inhibition of gastric motility associated with anxiety, and therefore will continue to eat as much when frightened as when calm.

Schachter and his colleagues administered a so-called 'taste test' to obese and non-obese college students under conditions

of low and high fear (Schachter *et al.*, 1968). The fear manip-
ulation was that subjects were told that during the experiment
they would be given electric shocks, mild in the low fear
condition, and strong in the high fear condition. In response to
high anxiety the normal weight subjects ate less than when
calm, while the obese subjects ate a little more (not significantly
so) in the anxious than in the calm condition. However, the
study has not been consistently replicated, and although it
suggests a feasible explanation for eating by obese people under
conditions of anxiety, the effect of fear on eating was not a
strong one and the results do not explain the powerful urge to
eat when anxious actually described by many people.

The Psychosomatic Hypothesis

An alternative explanation for overeating in obese people,
particularly in response to anxiety, is offered by the Psychosomatic Hypothesis. This is contradictory to Schachter's
theory as it bases itself on the assumption that obese people eat
in response to stress, rather than simply continuing to eat
despite it. The theory is related to psychodynamic theories
which explain overeating as the outcome of or response to
emotional conflict. Kaplan and Kaplan (1957) have concluded
that as many as twenty-seven different meanings of overeating
have been proposed by different psychodynamic theorists, and
that virtually any emotional conflict may eventually result in
the overeating symptom. Examples of the widely diverse symbolic meanings which have been associated with obesity are: an
expression of hostility or defiance towards parental authority; a
means of obtaining affection and acceptance from others; an
expression of self-depreciation; a means of exhibitionism; a
way of possessing a desired sexual object such as a penis or a
breast (Glucksman, 1972). There is, however, no concrete
evidence for any of these ideas, and a more restrained,
common-sense view is encompassed by psychosomatic theory.
Thus Hilde Bruch (1974), herself a psychodynamically
oriented therapist, has moved away from specific psychodynamic ideas about, for example, orality. She has put forward the
thesis that the inability to eat normally stems from faulty early
learning experiences in fat people as it does in anorexics. In
effect, the aetiology she proposes for disorders both of under-

eating and of overeating is similar: the disorder is the result of consistently inappropriate responses to the infant's expression of his needs. On the one hand the child's needs are not recognised and are therefore in a sense denied or rendered insignificant, so that the child finds it increasingly difficult to differentiate its own needs and wants from those of others around it. On the other hand mothers of obese children may misinterpret their needs and use food as a universal pacifier. Hence the child does not learn to regulate its own food intake nor to deal with situations of stress, and may learn to experience stress and tension as a 'need to eat' instead of a cue for more appropriate emotions and behaviours such as anger or sadness.

The corollary to these ideas would be that obese people and overeaters should on the one hand eat more when anxious because they have learnt to do so and on the other hand should show a reduction in anxiety after eating.

None of the laboratory studies investigating the effects of arousal, anxiety, and fear on amount eaten has found that they have a significant effect (Spitzer and Rodin, 1981). In other words, obese people do not necessarily appear to eat more when made anxious. Where there was an effect, this could sometimes be accounted for by the obese eating more, sometimes by the normal weight eating less.

The suggested anxiety-reducing effect of eating has also not been demonstrated. For example, in the study by Schachter and his colleagues (1968) reported fear was reduced more for normal weight than for the obese subjects after eating the crackers, and in a later replication of the study too, even though the obese ate more than the non-obese, they did not rate their anxiety any lower after eating (McKenna, 1972).

The question arises as to why these studies should show so little, or so inconsistent an effect considering that clinically many obese people do claim to overeat when under stress. For example, anxiety and other stresses are often cited as reasons by obese people for not being able to keep to a diet (Leon and Chamberlain, 1973). In one study in which normal and over-weight college students were asked to monitor their food intake and prior mood over twelve days, the overweight students described themselves as more likely to snack subsequent to negative mood states than did the normal weight students (Lowe and Fisher, 1983).

97

One possible explanation for the lack of effect shown in fear-inducing laboratory studies is that the subjects were usually mildly overweight college students, whose experience may not accurately represent that of obese people who present for treatment at medical clinics. Another possible problem with the studies is that they all used different means of producing fear (Spitzer and Rodin, 1981). Most threatened people with electric shock, another told them, for example, that they would have problems with interpersonal relationships according to their results on a test of personality (Abramson and Wunderlich, 1972); another threatened subjects with taking large amounts of blood (McKenna, 1972).

Not only are the fear stimuli all different, but they are also very dissimilar to the kinds of experiences described by people who claim to eat in response to anxiety. One of the major ways in which they differ from common or garden everyday anxieties is that they are clearly definable, objective fears of the kind not frequently encountered as chronic worries in everyday life.

Joyce Slochower (1983) has taken the work in relation to anxiety as a cause of overeating further. She holds that the reason for the inconclusive nature of the findings of earlier studies is their use of contrived settings and minimally obese, largely male populations. She holds that the manipulations brought about 'controllable' as opposed to what she calls 'uncontrollable' anxiety. The psychosomatic hypothesis, however, implies that 'the experiential anxiety state that triggers eating may be diffuse, and its source frequently not understood by the obese person' (Slochower, 1976). She hypothesised that obese subjects would therefore be more likely to overeat in a situation where the cause of their anxiety was unspecified.

In a test of this hypothesis obese and normal weight subjects were led to believe that they were hearing feedback of their own heartbeats which were synthesized to sound either fast or slow. Snack food was made available, although of course the purpose of the experiment was disguised. Obese subjects did in fact eat more when they were not given a reason for their apparently high levels of arousal than when they were given a benign reason. Also, their anxiety was significantly reduced after eating. Normal weight subjects on the other hand ate more in the labelled than in the unlabelled high arousal condition. Dr

Slochower subsequently attempted a replication of this experiment, but in a real life situation. Moderately obese and normal weight students were tested during and after their examination period, a time of uncontrollable anxiety owing to the unpredictable nature of the tests and the importance of these in the students' futures. The obese students ate more than twice as much during the final examination period as when the examinations were over, and there was a significant correlation between self-reported anxiety, loss of control and eating at both sessions (Slochower *et al.*, 1981).

On the one hand therefore, there is some evidence that obese people are reactive to their internal, emotional state, which would fit in with the psychosomatic hypothesis. On the other hand the external hypothesis, for which there is some support, suggests that on the contrary, obese people are unresponsive to internal stimuli and hyper-responsive to external stimuli. In an attempt to resolve this apparent contradiction, Dr Slochower went on to examine the possible interaction between the two effects – anxiety and external responsiveness. In a further study she manipulated both anxiety level and cue salience (Slochower and Kaplan, reported in Slochower, 1983). The high anxiety condition consisted of telling people that they were to have a test of personality which would assess many characteristics including 'severe pathological tendencies'; in the low anxiety condition subjects were told they were about to have a test of personal taste, designed to detect, for example, 'preferences in art and music'. In both conditions, the subjects were made to feel that they could not control the outcome as the test would detect hidden traits. The food cues were 'M&M's', American small candied chocolates, like the English 'Smarties'. The salience of the M&M's was manipulated by means of the use of either a transparent or an opaque container. The obese group ate more when anxious than when calm, and their response was most marked when the available food was of high, as opposed to low, salience, in other words when they could see it better. In the low anxiety condition, however, their responses to high and low cue salience were no different.

The conclusion drawn from the experiment was that in studies which manipulate cue salience, obese subjects are more likely to respond to external cues under conditions of moderate to high anxiety.

The examination study was then repeated under conditions of high and low food salience and the joint effect of high food salience and anxiety on eating in obese people was confirmed. This might explain a previous finding of Slochower's that obese people claimed to eat less under conditions of high stress during the examination period because they needed to spend much of their time in the library where food was less available to them than at other times of the year.

Thus there is some evidence both that some obese people eat in response to external cues, in some situations; and that they eat in response to anxiety. There is less clear support for the notion that obese people eat in order to reduce anxiety.

Robbins and Fray (1980), however, have drawn an analogy between the phenomenon of stress-induced eating in humans and evidence from the animal literature. There are many examples in the ethology literature of stress-induced eating (Morley *et al.*, 1983). For example, animals may eat in between bouts of fighting or when frustrated during courtship behaviour. Attention has been drawn to this phenomenon by work with animals in the laboratory, and specifically by the finding that rats respond to the stressor of having their tails pinched, by eating (Rowland, Antelman and Seymour, 1976). Researchers involved in this work point out that the response does not serve to reduce anxiety, but that the eating response may be just one of a range of responses to the activating effects of stress. Robbins and Fray (1980) suggest that it may be learnt in the way that compulsive behaviour may be learnt, also a behaviour which, contrary to previous opinion, has been shown not to reduce anxiety.

There are, then, many different stimuli that may produce eating in obese people. However, it is clear from a survey of what we do know that we cannot generalise about the psychological causes of overeating and hence of overweight for all obese people. It is likely that there are some effects which have a role in the initiation and perhaps maintenance of obesity in some people, possibly in combination with other, physiological or genetic, predisposing factors. Not all obese people respond in the same way, however, to environmental stimuli, to food itself, or to psychological stressors.

There may be a style of eating and responses to environmental phenomena which for some people enhance a tendency to grow fat and stay that way. On the other hand, it is important to be more than a little wary of extrapolating from the results of experiments using samples mainly of moderately obese students to explain the behaviour of moderately to grossly overweight people who present at clinics requesting help with weight reduction and/or modification of uncontrollable eating habits.

8 Overeating and people of normal weight

The phenomenon of overeating is not confined to fat people. In studies examining the determinants of overeating it has become increasingly clear that in some situations many people can be induced to overeat, be it in response to availability, high palatability, or even 'stress'.

Emphasis has shifted in the last few years from the psychology of the obese person *per se* to that of the overeater, be it the thin, the fat, or the normal weight overeater. This shift has occurred as the phenomenon of self-confessed overeating by people of normal weight has caught the attention of the medical and psychological world and even of the popular press.

In 1979, Gerald Russell, specialising in the treatment of anorexia nervosa, described a series of thirty patients most of whom had a history of anorexia nervosa, but whose weight was currently within normal limits. These (mainly) women experienced powerful and uncontrollable urges to overeat, which they alternated with periods of abstinence; like anorexics, they had a 'morbid fear of fatness' and in order to stabilise their weights they had developed the habit of vomiting or purging, or both. Russell called this syndrome 'bulimia nervosa' (Russell, 1979).

The syndrome, or variations on the syndrome, has also been named 'bulimarexia' (Boskind-Lodahl and White, 1978), 'dietary chaos syndrome' (Palmer, 1979), 'subclinical anorexia nervosa' (Button and Whitehouse, 1981), 'abnormal normal weight control syndrome' (Crisp, 1981) and just 'bulimia'.

Since Russell's paper, the literature on binge-eating in normal weight people has grown, as more workers have described it and variations on the syndromes bulimia or bulimia nervosa, and the results of surveys have begun to suggest that the problem of binge-eating in people of normal weight may exist on a fairly wide scale.

Epidemiology of binge-eating

Wardle (1980) in a survey of 68 medical students, reported that the 30 women admitted binge-eating on average at least four times a month and the 38 men at least twice a month. Binge-eating in this context was defined as 'eating lots of food even when not hungry', so it is important to note that binge-eating when defined in this way is possibly something that we all do from time to time. In another study of 100 students 40 per cent reported that they binge-ate, defined as eating because of a particular mood and when not hungry, at least three times a month (Edelman, 1981). Both in this study and in another in which 20 undergraduates were asked whether they 'engage in periods of uncontrollable excessive overeating' there was no correlation between the degree of binge-eating and current weight (Wolf and Crowther, 1984).

It is questionable whether binge-eating represents of itself a new medical or psychological problem: it is possible that the habit of occasionally eating a too large meal or of eating a packet of biscuits or more is a habit newly developed in this century, but an alternative explanation is that 'binge-eating' is merely an old habit that has become a new focus for introspection in a weight-conscious world.

Stricter criteria for defining binge-eating as a disorder appeared in the 1980 version of the Diagnostic and Statistical Manual of the American Psychiatric Association (DSM III). Their definition requires that episodic binge-eating be accompanied by an awareness that the eating pattern is abnormal, fear of not being able to stop eating voluntarily, and depressed mood and self-depreciating thoughts following the eating binges. Three out of five additional features must be present. These are: consumption of high-calorie food during a binge; inconspicuous eating during a binge; termination of binge episodes by abdominal pain, sleep, social interruption or self-induced vomiting; repeated attempts to lose weight by strict dieting, vomiting or purging; and frequent weight fluctuations of ten pounds or more.

Using these criteria, Halmi and her colleagues surveyed 355 college students and found that as many as 13 per cent of respondents experienced all the major symptoms. Only two thirds of the students surveyed had returned the questionnaire completed but even so this result suggested that the problem could be fairly widespread, at least among students (Halmi *et al.*, 1981).

In England this conclusion was borne out by the response to a magazine survey initiated by Fairburn and Cooper (1982). Through an article in a popular women's magazine in 1980, Dr Fairburn invited women who used vomiting as a means of controlling their weight to write to him. He received over 1,000 replies, which suggested that binge-eating is not confined to students. He then sent questionnaires to 800 of the women, and of the 669 returned, after excluding all those who probably suffered from anorexia nervosa, the authors concluded that 83 per cent fulfilled Russell's criteria for bulimia nervosa (stricter than the DSM III criteria in that they require the presence of purging).

Most of what is known about bulimia is in fact culled from questionnaires returned by or interviews with people, mainly women, who select themselves in response to the above kind of survey or who present for treatment or write for advice to centres known for their work on the disorder. In this way, Johnson and his colleagues in Chicago, for example, have had requests for help from several hundred women who have in turn provided information about the disorder (Johnson *et al.*, 1983).

In order to find out more about the prevalence of bulimia in the population as a whole, it is of course important to survey in a more random fashion, and researchers who have been able to do this have produced some interesting findings. In 1983, Cooper and Fairburn reported on the results of a survey they conducted of several hundred consecutive attenders at a family planning clinic in England. In this way they were able to obtain a fairly wide cross-section of the population – women up to the age of forty who use birth control. Of the 369 women who completed their questionnaire, more than a quarter reported ever having experienced a binge, defined as 'an episode of uncontrollable excessive eating', 20 per cent in the last two months. One fifth of the women reported that they had an eating problem. Eleven women had induced vomiting in the last two months, and the authors concluded that seven subjects, 1.9 per cent of the sample, currently fulfilled Russell's criteria for bulimia nervosa.

In another attempt to look beyond the studies of students and subjects who refer themselves, Pope and his colleagues distributed questionnaires to over 300 women shoppers in a suburb of Boston (Pope *et al.*, 1984). Of the sample, 10.3 per cent met DSM III criteria for a lifetime diagnosis of bulimia, in that they had experienced the symptoms in the past, and 4.6 per cent was actively bulimic. When the authors defined bulimia more narrowly as binge-eating at least once a week and vomiting or purging, then only four of the respondents could be described as actively bulimic and another five remitted, which suggests a percentage remarkably close to that found by Cooper and Fairburn (1983).

It is possible, then, that at any one time up to 2 per cent of women up to the age of forty years may be experiencing serious problems with controlling their eating.

Few men appear to suffer from bulimia. In one eating disorders clinic in Minnesota, only three men were seen during a three-year period in which 300 women presented themselves for treatment (Mitchell and Goff, 1984). Male bulimics who do present have features similar to those of women (Pope *et al.*, 1986); but although there is evidence that some men are as prone to the occasional bout of overeating as women are (Wardle, 1980), there is no reason to suspect that men suffer as frequently with bulimia as do women.

The average age of women affected is consistently suggested to be around 24 years, with a range of 18 to 34 years. The average age of onset of the disorder is around 16 to 18 years, but it may affect girls as young as 11 years (Pyle *et al.*, 1981) and women in their 40s (Chiodo and Latimer, 1983) although it is rare for the disorder to begin after the age of 30.

The consistent discrepancy between the age of people known now to have bulimia and the age of onset of the disorder appears to be due to the length of time that elapses before people seek treatment, which averages around five and one half years according to several authors (Johnson and Berndt, 1983; Pyle *et al.*, 1981; Abraham and Beumont, 1982); and may be as long as twenty-three years (Pope *et al.*, 1984). Many people never do seek help for the disorder. Pyle, reporting on patients in a psychiatric outpatient clinic, found that most people did not know anyone else with the problem and feared that if they asked for help they would be thought 'weird'. In response to Fairburn and Cooper's questionnaire study only just over half the sample thought they needed help but even so only one third of the whole group had ever mentioned their problem to a doctor and as few as 2.5 per cent were currently receiving any treatment. While it is true that many people who are referred to hospital outpatient clinics for 'weight' problems are in fact of normal weight, many people who visit their general practitioners may not be taken seriously as having a problem if they look normal and are of normal weight.

The nature of bulimia

It is fairly difficult to define what binge-eating in bulimia actually consists of, partly because what constitutes a great deal of food is so subjective a matter, and partly because a binge, by its very nature, is unobservable. A binge may be a short, discrete episode of eating very high calorie food, or an episode lasting anything from fifteen minutes to several hours. In Pyle's survey (1981) of thirty-four patients in an outpatient clinic, he asked ten patients to keep records of their binge-eating. The median duration of a binge was one hour, and the longest time reported was eight hours. The time between binges also appears to vary a great deal. Some binge-eaters may binge in several, up to perhaps six, discrete episodes in one day (Abraham and Beumont, 1982). Between one quarter and one half of binge-eaters asked about how often they binge-eat do it at least once a day, another 30–40 per cent between one and several times a week. Some people describe themselves as experiencing one long continuous binge from getting up in the morning to going to bed at night, for days, perhaps even weeks, at a time. Abraham and Beumont noted that the longer people had been binge-eating, the longer were their binge episodes.

The DSM III criteria suggest that bulimics eat rapidly, but while people with the disorder newly acquired eat fast, often without tasting the food after the initial intake, people who have been doing it for several years describe eating more slowly, often tasting small morsels of different foods one after the other, preparing the next food item while eating the first. Many binges are in fact planned. Three quarters of Abraham and Beumont's sample admitted to planning binges. This may involve buying food in, preparing and sometimes hoarding it. Some bulimics describe feelings of intense panic if they are unable to get hold of their favourite food items, and may even go out at night or at inconvenient times in search of them if they are not available at home.

The kind of food chosen is invariably food not eaten at other times, high in calorie, often easily and quickly digestible – custard, puddings, porridge. Most bulimics describe binge-eating in private, usually at home, rarely in public. If food has to be bought, then some binge-eaters may use different shops on different occasions in order to avoid potential embarrassment. Usually binge-eating takes place at home, but sometimes elsewhere, for example some people describe eating in the privacy of their car, or while walking along the street. If a great deal of food is eaten at home, this may be covertly replaced, although once other people have found out about it, many patients admit to it and will occasionally binge-eat in the presence of family members (Abraham and Beumont, 1982).

Most bulimics describe binge-eating as beginning late in the day, for example after returning from work or school (Pyle *et al.*, 1981; Mitchell *et al.*, 1981). They have difficulty in eating regular meals when not binge-eating, and difficulty in knowing when they are 'full' at the end of a 'normal' meal. This may explain Abraham and Beumont's finding that for a third of patients binge-eating is confined to certain times of day and the finding that binges are often temporally associated with mealtimes (Johnson and Larson, 1982).

The number of calories consumed may vary – between a reported 1,000 calories per binge to as many as 55,000 (Johnson *et al.*, 1982). The type of food eaten at other times, however, may be fairly limited. Weiss and Ebert (1983) questioned fifteen bulimics and fifteen control subjects who had never experienced an eating disorder. They found that control subjects ate on average almost twice as many times in a day as did bulimics and also a greater variety of foods, whereas the bulimics tried to keep planned meals to low-calorie items, such as cottage cheese, diet crackers, and salads.

After a binge, some bulimics simply run out of steam, others stop only when their stomach is distended to the point of discomfort; yet others stop only in response to social interruption. Often the binge-eating can be enjoyable, at least at first, but in general bulimics describe feelings of immense guilt, and self-disgust. Some try very hard to resist the behaviour, looking for alternatives to do – leaving the house, telephoning friends.

For many the binges alternate with up to several days of starving, during which sufferers feel strong and in control, only to grow hungry again and start to binge-eat once more.

This is where for some people vomiting and purging become essential to the behaviour. Many bulimics originally make the discovery perhaps after one occasion of being sick after a particularly heavy binge, or in association with a gastro-intestinal upset, and learn to use vomiting in the future as a means of getting rid of unwanted calories and of giving themselves the chance to 'start afresh'. Probably half the sufferers who use vomiting in this way had the idea themselves, but another quarter claim to have heard the idea from the media and another 17.4 per cent from friends and relatives (Fairburn and Cooper, 1982).

Not all bulimics use vomiting or laxatives as a way of controlling their weight, and this is where the problem arises with the definition of the disorder. According to DSM III criteria, vomiting is one of several conditions which may indicate the presence of the disorder, whereas according to Russell (1979), it is an essential criterion and therefore of course the prevalence of vomiting or purging in any one sample of patients is to some extent determined by the method with which the sample is chosen. Where the presence of vomiting is not an essential criterion of selection, its presence may occur in from anywhere between 12 and 80 per cent of sufferers (Stangler and Prinz, 1980; Johnson et al., 1982). Most people learn to do it at first by using their fingers or perhaps a toothbrush to induce the gag reflex. Thereafter, some learn to do it spontaneously. Unlike anorexics, some sufferers may continue with the habit for years without detection by family or friends – and even when detected some are able to evade explanation with the story that they have eaten something that disagreed with them.

Purging in some form or other usually has its onset about one year after the onset of binge-eating. Most people who use it describe an immense sense of relief on its discovery, as this means that each episode of binge-eating can be wiped out and the sufferer can convince herself that she is beginning again with a clean slate. Vomiting does not appear to occur as frequently as binge-eating. As a result of Fairburn and Cooper's magazine survey, over half the respondents confessed to vomiting at least once a day, 17 per cent at least once a week, and nearly 40 per cent of these said that they did it in total secrecy.

Some bulimics who vomit several times a day may vomit after a binge and then start again, going through the same sequence several times in a day. For some people the vomiting becomes a carefully worked-out process where the plan to binge-eat depends upon the subsequent availability of the opportunity to vomit. 'I can be sick tonight, so I can eat . . .' Russell (1979) describes one of his patients as being able when necessary to desist from overeating and vomiting for weeks at a time, but only by reducing her intake of food to 800 calories per day. The vomiting itself may be planned to such an extent that the sufferer will use 'markers' – brightly coloured food to start off with, so that she is able to tell from the colour of the vomitus when she has managed to rid herself of everything eaten. Some people even use washing-out techniques, drinking water and vomiting again until the vomit is clear (Abraham and Beumont, 1982).

Many people use laxatives as a means of purging, some in addition to vomiting, some when the opportunity to vomit is less available. Figures for the number of people who use laxatives as a means of purging vary from around one third to two thirds of bulimics. Laxatives are used less frequently than is vomiting. About a quarter of sufferers may take laxatives as well as vomiting daily (Johnson *et al.*, 1982) and usually in several times the recommended dose.

Some people use diuretics instead or in addition. It is possible that in some respects the effects are similar, as some patients describe the effect of the laxatives as dehydrating, serving to make them feel less 'bloated', and immediately thinner as a consequence. Contrary to the beliefs of most bulimics, laxatives may not in any case get rid of many unwanted extra calories. In a study planned to investigate this, Bo-Linn and his colleagues cleansed the entire gastro-intestinal tracts of two bulimic and two normal women prior to a test meal and again twelve to twenty-four hours later. They gave laxatives to the bulimics which caused five to six litres of diarrhoea in a twenty-four hour period. Calorie absorption decreased by only about 200 calories over the 1,500 to 2,000 taken in. The authors concluded that by the time chyme and digestive juices have traversed the stomach and small intestine and reached the colon, almost all the ingested foods that will be absorbed have been absorbed already, and any apparent weight loss is largely through dehydration (Bo-Linn *et al.*, 1983). These conclusions are supported by the finding that purgers in fact weigh more on average than do vomiters, but that they eat less (Lacey and Gibson, 1985).

Many bulimics also use exercise as a means of dissipating energy, in the same way that anorexics do: but in general bulimics do not necessarily exercise any more than do normal people (Cooper *et al.*, 1984).

This whole process of binge-eating and purging of course takes a tremendous toll on the physical well-being of sufferers. Three quarters of the 500 patients surveyed by Johnson and his colleagues in an eating disorders centre in Chicago noticed a change in their physical health. Tiredness, stomach disorders, dry skin and hair were among symptoms noticed (Johnson *et al.*, 1983). In an earlier study 20 per cent of their subjects reported amenorrhoea, and 50 per cent current menstrual irregularity (Johnson *et al.*, 1982). Pyle, in his survey, noted that twenty-six out of thirty-four subjects had had at least one episode of amenorrhoea for three months or more.

The vomiting itself predisposes people to metabolic complications. Potassium, chloride and hydrogen ions are lost in vomitus and symptoms include muscle weakness, constipation, headache, palpitations, abdominal pain and easy fatiguability (Harris, 1983). Oedema and possible kidney dysfunctions have also been reported and a predisposition to cardiac arrhythmias. The vomiting can also cause a range of other problems from sore throat, reported by many patients, and swollen salivary glands, to the more rare rupture of the oesophagus. The frequent presence of vomitus in the mouth can cause tooth enamel to dissolve, and many bulimics have sensitive teeth or develop an increase in dental caries due to the increased sugar intake. Some vomiters, aware that their teeth can suffer, take the extra precaution of visiting the dentist more frequently to check on this.

The amenorrhoea has been thought in the past to be a function of low weight, but as Crisp has pointed out, famines in the third world do not appear to significantly impair reproductive function (Crisp, 1981). Certainly for the high percentage of bulimics who have irregular periods or none at all this appears to be related to the abnormal eating behaviour itself. One patient of mine commented that her periods always seemed to stop whenever her bingeing and purging were at their worst.

The causes of bulimia

There is no clear answer as yet to the question of why the cycle of binge-eating and purging should arise in normal weight, apparently ordinary people.

The most common initial cause cited is a period of increased concern about body weight, sometimes leading to fairly stringent dieting in between one third and two thirds of sufferers. The one consistent major finding of all studies of bulimics is that most of them feel fat all of the time, and most have an ideal desired weight of at least some 10 per cent below their current weight, and lower than the ideal weight of non-bulimics. Such is their concern, that some may weigh themselves several times a day, while others assiduously avoid the scales for fear of what they might see. Usually bulimics also have fairly low self-esteem and a low level of satisfaction with their body image. The lower the satisfaction in these areas the greater the likelihood of binge-eating (Wolf and Crowther, 1983).

While many binge-eaters consider themselves overweight, they have not necessarily been either considerably overweight or considerably underweight in the past. Between 30 and 40 per cent of bulimics have, according to their own report in various surveys, been more than 20 per cent overweight in the past, and perhaps one quarter have been more than 25 per cent below average weight, possibly satisfying the criteria for anorexia nervosa. Some people may have reached weights in both categories of course, and Abraham and Beumont (1982) have noted that while some of their outpatients varied between high and normal weights, others moved between low and normal.

One factor very commonly associated with the onset of binge-eating and bulimia is that of 'stress'. For around 40 per cent of bulimics the onset of binge-eating is associated with life-style changes or with difficulty experienced with particular emotions such as depression, loneliness or boredom (Yates and Sambrailo, 1984; Johnson et al., 1982). The life-style changes cited may be changes at work, loss or separation from close relatives or friends, or conflict with family or spouse. The concept of 'stress' is itself of course a very difficult one to define ol to be specific about, and it may be useful to remember that probably the changes and conflicts noted are changes and conflicts as experienced by the person reporting them. In an albeit very small survey bulimics reported no greater number of stressful life events such as divorce, separations, house moves, or deaths than did normal subjects (Weiss and Ebert, 1983). Yet in a questionnaire survey comparing bulimic students and normal controls, there appeared to be a relationship between the amount of stress the bulimics believed themselves to have experienced and the severity of their binge-eating (Wolf and Crowther, 1983).

The binges themselves are reported to be triggered by a variety of negative moods and events; for example feeling sad and unhappy, feeling bored, anxious or tired, thinking about food, craving particular foods, feeling hungry, drinking alcohol, eating a meal in a restaurant, going out with a member of the opposite sex. Any of these either alone or in combination may lead to a binge episode.

Psychopathology of binge-eaters

If people who binge-eat and vomit admit to moods as triggers, then the question arises as it does with overweight people as to whether bulimics differ psychologically from other people.

Certainly in terms of behaviour alone, many bulimics exhibit characteristics that would be considered abnormal. A high proportion of bulimics admit to stealing; in American studies the figure is about two thirds (Weiss and Ebert, 1983; Pyle *et al.*, 1981), whereas in England only one third of a group referred to a psychiatrist admitted to stealing (Fairburn and Cooper, 1984). Food is usually the first item stolen and most continue only with this, giving the reason that they cannot afford to buy all the food needed to support the binge-eating, while some people have admitted to going on to other items such as clothes (Pyle *et al.*, 1981). Bulimics usually describe themselves as feeling terribly guilty about the stealing and often by the time they are questioned about it they have stopped doing it altogether. One person out of an English group of thirty-five people had previously had a problem with drug dependency but with a similar number in an American group nearly a quarter admitted to previous dependency (Pyle *et al.*,

1981) and in a group of fifteen bulimic students significantly more people had used cocaine, amphetamines and barbiturates than in a control group. Some bulimics also use slimming tablets as a means of weight control and these too may become addictive and hence a problem in themselves. In a survey of over 100 consecutive bulimics who presented to an eating disorders clinic in Minnesota, 30 per cent were using stimulant drugs daily, 9 per cent were taking sedatives, and 8 per cent were taking caffeine pills (Hatsukami et al., 1984).

This kind of behaviour raises the question of whether binge-eaters are psychologically different from other people. If so, then do all binge-eaters share the same psychopathology? These issues raise a third, perhaps stickier issue of what might underlie this behaviour and the moods and attitudes associated with it.

The personality of the bulimic has often been described as impulsive and neurotic; doctors and other health workers and dieticians alike are frequently rendered helpless by the intensity with which bulimics appear to be asking for help on the one hand and the apparent lack of 'motivation' with which they are able to adhere to suggested treatment on the other. Several researchers have attempted to draw some conclusions about the personality of the bulimic. The problem, as always in the sphere of personality assessment, is that every researcher uses different measures. Given this qualification, fairly common findings are that bulimics describe themselves as being low in self-esteem compared with other people, high in anxiety, lower in the feeling of control over their own lives, and unhappy with their body image (Grace et al., 1985). In one study negative attitudes to food and eating, extent of satisfaction with body image and level of self-esteem were the best predictors of binge-eating (Wolf and Crowther, 1983).

Nevertheless, there are many people who binge-eat, who hold down perfectly good jobs, and do well in them, and whose social lives appear to be unaffected by the behaviour, apart from the need to make time to eat and to find the privacy where necessary to vomit. In a survey among college women, Thompson and Schwartz (1982) compared those with 'anorexic-like' behaviour in terms of their high scores on the Eating Attitudes Test with problem-free women. They found that although the anorexic-like women were preoccupied with food and eating, this did not, according to their own reports, affect their academic performance or their social lives which were just as 'normal' as those of problem-free women. However, in another survey where the stricter criteria of DSM III were used, the authors concluded that bulimic women were less well adjusted in relation to work, social, leisure and family activities than were a normal community sample. More than two thirds of their clients reported that their eating difficulties had a very large influence over how things went in their daily activities and, in relation to interpersonal relationships (Johnson et al., 1983).

It is feasible that the 20 per cent of adult women who may be binge-eating regularly are fairly 'normal' in most respects. Some of the smaller group of people who satisfy DSM III criteria, however, and in particular those who satisfy Russell's criteria which necessitate the presence of frequent vomiting, clearly have serious problems. In the course of their disorder, their socioeconomic and family backgrounds, and in their response to the Eating Attitudes Test, many bulimics do not differ from the bulimic group of anorexics (Herzog and Norman, 1985). As with many anorexics also, several bulimics could be classified as having a psychiatric disorder.

Certainly there can be no underestimation of the degree of distress caused by the disorder of bulimia itself: 50 per cent of bulimics in one survey confessed to having had thoughts of suicide, and nearly 20 per cent had actually attempted it, a quarter of these seriously (Johnson et al., 1983). In another study as many as 70 per cent admitted to suicidal ideas (Abraham and Beumont, 1982).

More than two thirds of the women who responded to the Oxford magazine survey scored above the threshold on the General Health Questionnaire, which is a test of general psychological disturbance or malaise (Fairburn and Cooper, 1982). At the same time, across several studies, authors have described bulimics as rating themselves as significantly more sad, lonely, weak and irritable than other people, with wider oscillations between states of happiness and sadness than others (Johnson and Larson, 1982) and frequently more depressed in general (Weiss and Ebert, 1983). Over half the patients who presented themselves for treatment at one eating disorders clinic rated themselves as moderately to severely depressed on the Beck Depression Inventory (Hatsukami et al., 1984).

Several authors have concluded that up to 80 per cent of bulimics would qualify either now or in the past for a diagnosis of major depressive disorder according to both the American and British systems (Fairburn and Cooper, 1984; Pope and Hudson, 1984). Other estimates are more conservative, with less than 20 per cent of people surveyed having sought psychiatric treatment in the past (Hatsukami et al., 1984). The presence of depression raises the question of whether the disorder comes first, and leads to the depression, as well it might, or whether in fact the disorder itself is a manifestation of a so-called 'affective disorder'. The relevance of the sequence of events to some researchers is that if indeed bulimia is a manifestation of depression, then it should be possible to treat it medically in the same way, with the same drugs.

In a study in England, thirty-six subjects diagnosed as having bulimia nervosa were rated as to their level of depression and anxiety at the beginning of treatment and subsequently at regular intervals (Johnson-Sabine et al., 1984). Their mean initial scores on the Hamilton Rating Scale for depression fell within the range of mild affective disturbance. Self-rated mood was consistently worse on the first day of a binge for most subjects compared to the day before and worse still when patients were vomiting as well. The authors concluded that the negative mood changes associated with bulimia nervosa do not constitute a major mood disorder, and that the behaviour comes first, followed by a change in mood. From a clinical point of view, this fits in to some extent with what some people say, but one would also expect a drop in mood prior to the behaviour, as so many people describe depressed mood or some event with negative connotations as the trigger to binge-eating. Presumably such an effect could only be accurately picked up by the use of continuous or at least very regular mood monitoring.

Nevertheless the evidence is fairly equivocal, and other workers in the field conclude that it is the depression, in the form of a major affective disorder, that comes first.

Evidence which is claimed to support this theory comes from three sources. One of these is the presence of psychiatric illness in the families of bulimics. In Pyle's survey it was noted that 16 out of the 34 bulimics had at least one first degree relative who had been diagnosed as having depression. In Fairburn's study of out-patients referred to him, 29.4 per cent had a first degree relative who had also been treated by a psychiatrist, mostly for depression. Most of these reports were of course uncorroborated descriptions by the patients, but in a survey of 75 patients and their families Hudson and his colleagues concluded on the basis of interviews with 42 of the relatives and reports about the remainder that as many as 53 per cent of their patients had a father, a mother, or a sibling with a history of major depressive disorder. This they claim is higher than the incidence of depressive disorder in the relatives of depressed and schizophrenic patients in the population (Pope and Hudson, 1984). Nevertheless in a study in which family diagnoses were made blind to the probands' diagnosis, no greater prevalence of affective disorder was noted in the families of bulimics than in those of controls, on the basis of interviews with parents (Stern *et al.*, 1984).

What is not clear from these studies of course is how far the association where it exists is a causal one, the direct result of genetic influence, and how far it is the result of the bulimics and their depressed relatives being exposed to similar environmental influences.

There has also been some suggestion that bulimics respond physiologically in similar ways to people with clinical depression. Some bulimics have a shortened REM latency which compares with that of depressed patients (Katz *et al.*, 1984); they also respond in a similar way to depressed people to the dexamethosone suppression test and the thyrotropin releasing hormone stimulation test. These responses could of course result from the effects of stress itself but the response appears to be the same whatever the degree of binge-eating, and even occurs in people not currently binge-eating. However the evidence cannot be taken as conclusive, as the meaning of the two tests is not yet clear and responses to them could merely be non-specific reactions to any kind of stress.

A third factor which suggests that bulimia may be a major affective disorder is in relation to its treatment. There have been several treatment trials using anti-depressant drugs. Some binge-eaters binge less or stop altogether in response to anti-depressant drug therapy, and this area will be further discussed in more detail in Chapter 12.

There is some evidence, therefore, of a relationship between bulimia and affective disorder, just as there may be a relationship between anorexia nervosa and the affective disorders.

But how far it is useful to view bulimia or bulimia nervosa as an affective disorder akin to depression but with different symptoms will clearly depend on how far the evidence stands up to further research, and also upon how far it becomes practicable to treat both disorders in the same way.

Behavioural aspects of binge-eating

A more behavioural explanation of bulimia and vomiting is related to the idea that the behaviour comes to be rewarding as a means of tension release. Exactly which aspects of the behaviour are most rewarding and therefore most likely to maintain the disorder are not clear, however. Some patients describe relief from tension and negative mood states during or immediately after binge-eating (Abraham and Beumont, 1982). Others describe a build-up of tension after binge-eating which may be relieved only by vomiting. Johnson and Larson (1982) conducted a study of the moods of binge-eaters using a time-sampling method in which they used electronic pagers to signal their subjects to fill in mood scales at random moments over a period of several days. The subjects' combined self-reports suggested that negative moods worsened during a binge but began, together with feelings of control and adequacy, to return to normal after a purge. On the basis of this study, the authors hypothesise that after some years the purging may become more rewarding than binge-eating and that some women may begin to binge-eat in order to experience the relief of a purge.

This would fit in with the experience of bulimics who declare to themselves during a day of stressful encounters at work or at home, 'Tonight I shall vomit, and so today I can eat.' Some bulimics do in fact claim to feel a relief after vomiting that is over and above the relief merely of having disposed of the contents of their stomach. The implication for treatment is that the vomiting itself would become the target for change, on the assumption that the binge-eating which has become of secondary importance will be reduced as a consequence. It is difficult, though, for most bulimics to separate the experience of the desire to binge from that of the decision to vomit, and to seek out anything other than a cure for the bulimia in which the bingeing and purging are closely linked. Nevertheless the issues surrounding the maintenance of the disorder will only be elicited as behaviour therapy becomes a more refined tool in relation to its treatment.

Cultural determinants of binge-eating

Another very different way of looking at the disorder is from the sociological, historical point of view. The fact that bulimia has become of interest to the medical and psychological world only since the late 1970s suggests that there may be some cultural factor at work, at least in relation to the way in which the disorder manifests itself and is maintained, if not in its aetiology.

It is probably not an overestimate of the problem to note that many women see themselves as fatter than they should be, and that this attitude has a basis in the reality of a general attitude to women which means that they are often denied access to social privilege on the basis of their physical appearance (Wooley and Wooley, 1980). In this atmosphere it is common for a slim woman at a social gathering to glance conspiratorially at another while accepting an item of food and mutter, 'I'll be good tomorrow.' Implicit in the communication is that to eat certain foods, to not keep to a reducing diet for a woman in particular is generally perceived as inadvisable, whereas to deprive oneself of good foods and to exhibit 'will-power' and 'self-control' is intrinsically good and seemly, and to be admired.

It is in this atmosphere where thinness is to be praised and coveted and hence by implication also the process of dieting, that many writers believe the chronic dieter is nurtured by society to a stage in which she is repeatedly 'on a diet', staying at a health farm, or on a new exercise regime.

The Wooleys (1982) even go so far as to suggest that some diets might teach women to develop a kind of anorexia nervosa as a cure for overweight. In a comment on the *Beverley Hills Diet* (Mazel, 1981) they suggest that the encouragement, for example, to eat only fruit all day to compensate and allow for the possibility of days of binge-eating is akin to marketing anorexic behaviour. To eat in large amounts one day and starve the next or to eat so as to create a laxative effect, is to do as the anorexic or the bulimic does. This kind of eating behaviour, say the Wooleys 'reveals a degree of desperation heretofore unknown'. Yet the exhortation to starve in order to lose weight fast, to get rid of that flab for the winter, the summer, Christmas, the New Year, is commonly seen in the women's pages of the daily newspapers. The diet advised is always new, always guaranteed to lose several pounds a week usually by taking in a very small number of calories, often in strange culinary combinations, for a short period of time.

In this context, say the feminist writers, the development of compulsive eating behaviour is a natural corollary to the experience of pressure to be thin and hence culturally acceptable. One proponent of this view is Susie Orbach whose book *Fat is a Feminist Issue* has been welcomed by many women (Orbach, 1978). According to Orbach, being fat or eating compulsively is a directed conscious or unconscious challenge to sex-role stereotyping and the culturally defined experience of womanhood (Orbach, 1978). In other words, a woman is expected by society to market herself as being available to men, marriage and motherhood. In the face of this pressure, exploited by advertising and the media, her desire to realise her potential as a person becomes of secondary importance in relation to her public image as an attractive female package. For some women compulsive eating develops as a way to avoid being 'marketed' in this way, a way to avoid competition with other women, and possibly the only way for a woman to defend herself against the powerlessness of her position in society *vis-à-vis* men.

Binge-eating and deprivation

Notwithstanding the likely cultural pressure on woman to diet, there may however be a simpler explanation for the binge-eating. In their studies of human starvation, Keys *et al.* (1950) found that men whether fat or thin became obsessed by thoughts and dreams of food. Food became the main topic of conversation and men who had previously had no special interest in food became interested in cookbooks and menus. After twelve weeks of semi-starvation the men were allowed to eat what they liked. In the thirteenth week many of them ate almost continuously. Some stated a preference for sweet or dairy products which lasted for some weeks and at least four out of the thirty-four subjects wanted to continue eating even when their stomachs were full. Several weeks later some of the men were continuing to eat what they described as 'prodigious' quantities of food and had gained weight, and some had put themselves on reducing diets.

These findings suggest the possibility that the experience of deprivation itself nurtures the desire to binge-eat, even after rehabilitation and after food has become freely available again.

Obese people, slim people on diets and starving anorexics all have in common the experience of long periods of deprivation and if indeed deprivation itself is a causative factor then this would explain the similarities across the three groups.

The deprivation involved might on the one hand have a physiological effect on the person deprived; it might on the other hand have an effect which was largely psychological, or a combination of both.

It is possible that the experience of being deprived of certain foods has a part to play in the phenomenon of bulimia where it is combined with diabetes. In recent years, several cases have been described in the literature of diabetics who binge-eat or who have bulimia or anorexia nervosa.

Control of insulin-dependent diabetes requires the patient to control his or her diet so that insulin requirements remain predictable and steady and so that weight gain is avoided (Hillard and Hillard, 1984). In order to avoid rapid rises in blood sugar, patients are usually encouraged to limit their intake of simple carbohydrates which in effect means snack or 'junk' foods. This means eating well-balanced regular meals, for some people counting calories or carbohydrates in order to maintain or reduce weight, and careful control over a list of 'forbidden foods'.

Knowledge about the long-term prognosis of the disease is fairly frightening to many people. Some patients admit to periods, especially at times soon after initial diagnosis, of behaving as though they did not have it, complying poorly with the treatment in the hope that if they ignore the disease it may go away. In a sense to binge-eat and purge is to do just this; bingeing on high carbohydrate food leads to hyperglycaemia due to excessive amounts of sugar, while purging leads to hypoglycaemia due to the relative excess of insulin. One way of controlling the binge-eating is to take less than the required amount of insulin as a way of losing sugar in the urine, and some sufferers, in particular anorectics, have been described as doing this despite the recognised long-term dangers (Szmukler and Russell, 1983). Others control the hyperglycaemia by taking more insulin, but as this leads to weight gain, a preferred method for some people is vomiting.

The symptoms of binge-eating followed by purging, the weight fluctuations, and the preoccupation with food are the same as those experienced by non-diabetic bulimics. The difference is that the behaviour is dangerous, at least in relation to the possible long-term complications resulting from long periods of fluctuating blood glucose levels; and that the diabetes itself may be used as a means of weight control. Diabetic patients who binge-eat or binge and purge have been described as having low self-esteem and as being more prone to depression than other diabetics. The symptoms characteristic of bulimics who have diabetes are fairly similar to those characteristic of other bulimics and it could be that the association between the two conditions is a chance one. On the other hand the development of bulimia is also fairly understandable in relation to the stress of having a chronic disease. The knowledge that one's body does not function exactly as it should without help could well for some people lead to a lowering of self-esteem and feelings of sadness, even depression. To 'rebel' against the necessary close control might for some people be a way to fight the disease, and such behaviour could no doubt be exaggerated by the involvement of a concerned family who might potentiate the dangers of the situation by its attempts to help.

The incidence of bulimia together with diabetes may be fairly high, as suggested by the reports of doctors who have observed several unexplained cases of poor control. Hudson et al. (1985), on the basis of a small survey of diabetic women, have suggested that the prevalence may equal or exceed that in age-matched populations of non-diabetic women. In another survey nearly 20 per cent of a sample of female diabetic adolescents suffered clinically significant eating and weight pathology and the authors suggested that eating disorders are at least twice as common in this group as in non-diabetic adolescents (Rodin et al., 1985). These findings would support the hypothesis that the diabetes may itself be a trigger for eating disorder.

The restraint hypothesis

Another way of looking at the phenomenon of overeating which has had important implications for the psychology of eating in general and eating in response to stress or deprivation in particular is in terms of the Restraint Hypothesis. The idea of 'Restraint' is consistent with the idea that normal weight as well as obese people may respond to external cues or eat in response to stress, but does not carry with it the notion that eating is necessarily anxiety reducing.

In 1975 Herman and Mack suggested that the distinction between external and internal responsiveness first proposed by Schachter might be explained by differences between dieters and non-dieters rather than by the difference between obese and normal weight people. Their hypothesis draws from the theory of Nisbett (1972) which implies that some obese people are underweight with regard to their biologically determined 'set-point'. As a result some obese people and also many normal weight people are in a state of chronic hunger due to having constantly to diet in order to keep their weight to a socially acceptable level. Herman and Mack called this phenomenon 'restraint', and they developed a scale to measure it on an individual basis. The scale has ten questions intended to tap responses in relation to weight history and the degree to which weight fluctuates, and level of concern about weight and dieting. At one extreme, the highest scoring person is one who diets frequently, whose weight fluctuates within short periods of time, and who spends a great deal of time thinking about food and feeling guilty about overeating. At the other extreme, with a low score on the scale, is the person whose weight rarely seems to fluctuate, who never diets, and does not worry about what she eats. Herman and Mack (1975) hypothesised that the restrained eaters, characterised by high scores on the scale, would resemble Schachter's (1968) obese subjects, failing to compensate for a preload by eating less subsequently, while unrestrained eaters would compensate appropriately, like Schachter's normal weight subjects. They measured response to a preload in two groups of normal weight subjects, the same in weight, but differentiated by their degree of restraint as measured by the scale. The unrestrained eaters compensated reasonably well for the preload but the restrained eaters responded in the opposite direction, and ate even more after a large preload of two milk shakes than after a smaller one (one milk shake).

This effect, called 'counter-regulation', was subsequently replicated in several experiments, usually on subjects of normal weight, and was found to be a better predictor of eating behaviour than was weight (Hibscher and Herman, 1977; Spencer and Fremouw, 1979).

There is little evidence that normal weight people are any better at short-term regulation than are obese people, which implies that eating behaviour may be controlled as often by cognitive cues as by physiological ones. Indeed some evidence had been suggested for the existence of cognitive factors in eating by previous work (Wooley, 1972; Nisbett and Storms, 1973). Both obese and normal weight subjects ate less after taking preloads labelled as high in calories than after preloads labelled as low calorie. Therefore Polivy (1976) went on to combine the work on cognitive factors in eating with the work on restraint. She categorised normal weight subjects on the basis of restraint, and assigned them to one of four conditions: where they were given either a high or a low calorie preload, and either true or false information about calorific value. Restrained subjects who perceived the preload as high in calories subsequently ate over 60 per cent more than those who perceived it as low in calories. Polivy points to the relevance of this finding in relation to dieters who may overeat following even a small slip in their diet and draws a parallel with an eating binge: the fact that the dieter believes she has overeaten is enough to trigger a binge. This is analogous to the experience of the person who says, 'I've ruined my diet now, I might as well give up and go on eating even more.' Even the anticipation of a dietary 'violation' may disrupt restraint. In one study where subjects were led to expect a milkshake, a salad or nothing after a cracker taste test, restrained eaters ate significantly more prior to the milkshake than did unrestrained eaters (Ruderman *et al.*, 1985).

The idea that restraint may be disrupted by both dietary and cognitive manipulations has been further explored in a series of experiments examining the response of restrained and unrestrained eaters to alcohol (Polivy and Herman, 1976). Alcohol itself did not in fact have the expected result of disinhibiting restrained subjects, but it did have the effect of producing counter-regulation when it was labelled as such; in other words restrained subjects ate more after they thought they had been given alcohol, a substance which everyone knows is disinhibiting.

Another phenomenon which has been examined in relation to restraint is that of eating more under conditions of emotional stress. Herman and Polivy (1975) found that restrained subjects ate more when made anxious; while unrestrained subjects ate less. Taking this idea further they administered the Restraint scale to twelve patients with a diagnosis of depression. The restrained patients said they had gained weight while depressed whereas the unrestrained patients reported themselves to have lost. Consistent with this finding are those of studies in which a depressed mood is induced in obese and non-obese students. In one study among self-confessed dieters, the depressed students ate nearly twice as much as the non-depressed students and this was true of all students whether obese or not (Baucom and Aiken, 1981). In other studies, with students of average weight classified as high or low restrained, the high restrained students responded to induced depressed mood by eating more in 'taste tests' than did subjects with low restraint scores or high restrained but undepressed subjects (Frost et al., 1982; Ruderman, 1985).

Restraint theory implies that this counter-regulation effect, the tendency for high restraint people to eat more when depressed, when they believe they have over-eaten or are about to do so, will occur in dieters of all weights. In other words, subjects who score high on the restraint scale are expected to respond as obese people do and vice versa.

However some researchers have found that unrestrained overweight people eat more than restrained overweight people in studies using preloads (Ruderman and Wilson, 1979; Ruderman and Christensen, 1983). Some people have suggested that this kind of inconsistency may rather be due to the psychometric properties of the Restraint scale itself than to real differences between obese and non-obese dieters. The Restraint scale includes questions about degree of overweight and weight fluctuations as well as about dietary concern, so it may be that overweight *per se* produces a higher score for some people than they might have if the questions were only about dietary concern. It has in fact been suggested that the dietary concern questions are better predictors of amounts eaten by people in a depressed mood than are the weight questions or the scale as a whole (Ruderman, 1985). A more recent scale has been devised by Stunkard which attempts to deal with this ambiguity. He based his new scale on the work of both Pudel and Herman. Pudel had proposed that normal weight people who fail to slow their rate of eating towards the end of a meal were 'latent obese' and on the basis of this he devised a scale similar to Herman's Restraint scale (Pudel *et al.*, 1975). Stunkard combined the items from the two scales and added some of his own to create a fifty-one-item questionnaire in which items contributed to one of three factors: 'cognitive restraint', 'tendency towards disinhibition' and 'perceived hunger' (Stunkard and Messick, 1985).

Whatever the relative merits of these available scales, still the possibility is emerging that there exists an eating style or possibly even a range of eating styles which mimic those customarily expected of obese people and which are based on a tendency to worry about weight and diet and to respond to many cognitive and emotional cues by eating, even overeating. As Herman and Polivy (1980) have pointed out, an interpretation of the combined data of studies using forced preloads, alcohol and induced anxiety or depression is in terms of their differential disinhibiting effects on restrained and unrestrained eating. In other words it is feasible not that eating produces relief from but that stresses of various types may result in a breakdown of self-control and hence to eating in some people. This is consistent with the evidence from the animal literature of eating in response to stress rather than as a means to reduce it (see Chapter 7).

Binge-eating in people of all weights may be fostered by a variety of pressures: cultural, environmental and intrapersonal. This is very different from the view of overeating as an affective disorder as it implies that eating and weight gain or bingeing and vomiting are phenomena which could be brought under environmental and cognitive control, given the right circumstances. Both views may be justifiable, in that just as externality may become more salient under conditions of stress (see Chapter 7), the phenomenon of restraint may be engendered and enhanced by clinical depression and vice versa.

Part III

Treatment of the eating disorders

Introduction

9

No one approach has yet proved exclusively effective in the treatment of either overeating or undereating. The degree of emphasis on either medical or psychological factors depends on the bias of the professionals who are offering treatment.

Decisions about treatment may rest upon whether the problem is seen as resulting from an interpersonal or from a sociocultural dilemma. If the symptoms of a disorder are interpreted as a scapegoat for contemporary problems in living, then the cure must be to develop more appropriate ways of coping. This implies that change must be effected through attitudinal or behavioural change, and treatment necessarily has a psychological bias.

If on the other hand, the disorder is viewed as having a largely physiological or biochemical basis then the natural corollary of this is treatment by means of pharmacotherapy or another medical intervention. The aetiology of most disorders of eating is, however, seldom so clear-cut as to lend itself to an unequivocal decision about treatment approach.

It is tempting for the patient to demand and for the physician to offer purely physical treatment for undereating or overeating. Yet the vagaries of patient compliance are such that outcome of treatment is rarely predictable. Overweight patients may beg for inpatient starvation, or for dental splinting; they may exhibit something akin to euphoria during weight loss, only to regain their lost weight after the restrictions have been removed. The problem of compliance is possibly more crucial in relation to anorexia nervosa. Forced to eat in order to escape from hospital, most anorexics will gain weight, only to lose it again on return to their previous circumstances.

It has become increasingly clear that even where medical treatment is offered for apparently medical problems, psychological factors have an immense part to play in the success of treatment and in the level of compliance with treatment. Preparation and recovery from surgery, dealing with pain, illness relating to cardiac problems, intestinal disorders, and diabetes – all are situations in which the importance of psychological factors in treatment has been increasingly appreciated in the past decade.

Overeating and undereating are truly psychosomatic disorders. It is very difficult to disentangle psychological from other factors, not least the physical problems inherent in being either overweight or underweight in itself. Moreover whatever the nutritional status of the individual, it is clear that both what we eat and whether we eat is always subject to a host of cognitive and environmental influences.

Psychologists and psychiatrists have for long addressed themselves to the problem of persuasion. Persuasion may take a variety of forms: from gentle exploration of motives and conflicts, to psychodynamic psychotherapy, to the 'magic' implied by hypnosis, or to coercion in the name of behaviour modification.

It is the rare treatment centre that does not now take psychological factors into account both in establishing the nature of the problem for the individual and in prescribing treatment. The question that remains is not whether psychological factors are important, but how far psychological treatments can be effective, either on their own, or in combination with medical and dietary treatments.

The emphasis of psychological treatment may be in the direction of exploring motivation to change as often as it addresses the question of how to effect change. This has provoked discussion of a new ethical problem – that of whether to treat at all. Such is the suffering of many obese people, for example, that unsuccessful treatment may frequently serve only to add to their suffering, to no avail. There is a view that a more humane approach might be to concentrate on helping the obese person, or equally the bulimic, to come to terms with her situation, to balance the potential of peace of mind against the health risks of remaining overweight or continuing to overeat.

Treatment of undereating and anorexia nervosa 10

Treatment of undereating itself is in many cases not appropriate. Treatment of anorexia can most often be effected through dealing with the underlying problem. Thus where psychiatric patients, for example, are anorexic as a result of depression, or in relation to a schizophrenic illness, the anorexia remits with treatment of the disorder. Similarly, patients with neurotic problems who may refuse to eat in public, for example, or for fear of choking, will eat normally again as soon as the phobia has responded to behaviour therapy or psychotropic medication.

In some cases a cure is more difficult. Cachexic patients with cancer present a major problem to the people looking after them. It has been suggested that one way of countering the problems of persuading cancer patients to eat is to make meals as enticing as possible by the way in which they are presented, to encourage a 'social' atmosphere around mealtimes by setting up meals with family or friends or at least with fellow patients, and possibly even adding some fine wines (Holland *et al.*, 1977).

Where anorexia nervosa is concerned, treatment is complicated by the difficulties inherent in understanding the nature of the disorder. Psychological, social and physiological factors are all considered to be of importance in the aetiology of anorexia nervosa, but there is no consensus about the relative importance of any one factor. This being so, there are differences in ways of restoring weight and the degree to which psychological treatments are used varies between specialist centres. Agras and Kraemer, who have reviewed all controlled treatment studies for anorexia nervosa up to 1982, have noted a change in emphasis of treatment since 1930 (Agras and Kraemer, 1984). Between 1930 and 1959 all patients were treated with medical therapy, consisting of hospitalisation plus confinement to bed, and possibly tube feeding sometimes with the addition of psychotherapy or family therapy. In the 1960s nearly 20 per cent of cases also received drug therapy; and behaviour modification was used in just under 20 per cent of cases. Since the 1970s drug therapy has been used in a quarter of all cases and behaviour modification or therapy in 45 per cent. It is also clear that even where a specific named treatment is offered, such as behaviour modification or psychotherapy, what is meant by these terms may differ greatly from one clinic to another.

The outstanding problem in assessing the efficacy of treatment for anorexia nervosa is that it is nearly impossible to compare the effects of treatment with no treatment at all. Possibly because of the serious nature of the disorder, there are no treatment trials in which treatment is compared with waiting list controls; and even patients who drop out of treatment are hard to follow up on the one hand and likely to have received additional treatment elsewhere on the other (Vandereycken and Pierloot, 1983).

More than thirty different therapies have been advocated for the treatment of anorexia nervosa but there are as yet no clear prognostic outcome studies which have demonstrated the particular advantage of any one treatment or combination of therapies over any other (Garfinkel and Garner, 1982).

In practice when writing about anorexia nervosa, most clinicians and research workers describe the treatments offered by themselves based on their own value judgments of what is available and on a considered opinion of what the patient needs (Russell, 1970, 1981; Andersen, 1985; Garfinkel and Garner, 1982).

What actually happens in terms of treatment then depends very much on the orientation of the physician or clinic to whom the sufferer is referred. Thus, for example, psychiatrists are more likely than physicians to use antidepressants, major tranquillisers and various forms of psychotherapy (Bhanji, 1979).

Medical treatment of anorexia nervosa

Most clinicians, physicians and psychiatrists alike, are agreed that a period of inpatient treatment in hospital is essential for the majority of anorexics in order to ensure weight gain. Most programmes advocate bedrest, sometimes with other restrictions also, such as no visitors; restrictions of the patient's freedom are gradually removed as she gains weight. The caloric value of diets offered is gradually increased each week until the patient may be taking 3,000 to 5,000 calories daily. On this kind of regime it may be possible to induce a gain of 28 pounds (12.7 kg) in eight weeks (Russell, 1970). In addition to medical treatments psychological treatments have traditionally been offered to a varying extent. For example, Crisp (1966) advocates that the patient spend four to five hours with the therapist during the first two weeks. During that time a formal psychiatric history is taken, the eating behaviour is explored, together with the patient's sexual activities, all in a fairly directive way, and the patient is then offered a possible explanation for her problem embodying the therapist's views of the nature of her disorder: for example that its metabolic effect is protecting her from sexual behaviour and feelings that formerly were intolerable to her. Help would be offered with these problems and the patient would then be seen by the therapist briefly once a day and for forty-five-minute sessions once a week. Russell (1981) places less emphasis on the psychotherapy aspect than on the aspect of skilled nursing care through which the nurses establish a relationship of trust with the patient who is asked to let them assume responsibility for choice of food and its amount. Supportive psychotherapy is offered 'if facilities permit' and prior to admission to specialist psychiatric units patients are persuaded to become inpatients through outpatient appointments (Russell, 1981).

Occasionally, if the anorexia is very severe, tube feeding has been used. However this has medical complications and is not advocated without absolute necessity (Garfinkel and Garner, 1982). More recently there have been reports of success using hyperalimentation or 'total parenteral nutrition', in which all essential nutrients are given to the patient by peripheral or central vein. This therapy has been used with patients who have failed previously to respond to anything else, and has produced weight gains of 5 to 12 kilograms (11 to 26 pounds) during hospitalisation (Maloney and Farrell, 1980). These gains are not necessarily greater than gains achieved by other treatments, however, as they are simply more rapid initially (Pertschuk *et al.*, 1981). Like tube feeding this treatment is also to be avoided if possible as there is a high risk of medical complications such as sepsis, vein thrombosis, liver toxicity and water overload (Maloney and Farrell, 1980).

Thus standard medical treatment usually consists of bedrest and nursing care alone, and is also supplemented by some form of psychotherapy or drug therapy.

Pharmacotherapy in anorexia nervosa

The use of chlorpromazine together with bedrest and a high calorie diet was advocated by Dally and Sargent (1966). The value of this drug was, according to Dally, its ability to allay fear in the patients and overcome resistance to eating. Between 1957 and 1962 they treated thirty patients with a combination of chlorpromazine and insulin in addition to the 'standard' treatment. They compared these patients with a group of eight treated with insulin alone and another group of twenty-seven patients treated previously in the 1940s and 1950s, with a 'standard' treatment of bedrest and high calorie diet. The authors claimed better weight gains and a shorter average time in hospital for the chlorpromazine treated patients. On three-year follow-up, however, the chlorpromazine group were doing no better than the other groups. Menstruation took twice as long to return on average in the chlorpromazine treated group and at follow-up nearly half of this group had developed bulimia compared to only 12 per cent in the usual care group. The addition of insulin had no effect on outcome, and although there are still some physicians who continue to use chlorpromazine, the use of insulin has not been continued. Chlorpromazine nevertheless also has its dangers – in terms of lowering the patient's blood pressure, and reducing body temperature (Garfinkel and Garner, 1982) and of increasing the risk of epileptic fits (Dally, 1969).

As an alternative way of reducing anxiety about eating, some people have advocated the use of minor tranquillisers (Bhanji, 1979; Garfinkel and Garner, 1982).

Another approach has been to use antidepressant medication, based on the hypothesis that many anorexics are depressed, or are in fact suffering from affective disorder (see Chapter 5). This approach is favoured particularly in the United States (Herzog, 1984a). Many researchers have claimed good results in terms of alleviation of depressed mood or weight gain using tricyclics (Moore, 1977; Needleman and Waber, 1977; Mills, 1976). However, the studies were not uniform or objective in their presentation of mood or weight data and cannot be conclusive. Lacey and Crisp (1980) completed a better controlled study, randomly assigned and double-blind, of chlomiprimene in sixteen anorexic patients who were also on hospital bedrest and receiving individual psychotherapy. The drug had no main effect on weight gain and all patients reached their target weights at a similar rate.

Another drug which has received some attention is lithium. In one study sixteen anorexics were randomly allocated to drug or placebo in a twenty-eight-day double-blind trial with both groups also participating in a behaviour modification programme (Gross et al., 1981). The drug had no effect on depressed mood, but the lithium group gained significantly more weight per month. However, the lithium group had in fact had a higher base-line calorie intake than the control group so it was not clear which factor was responsible for the faster weight gain. Moreover the authors themselves cautioned about the clinical dangers of using lithium in these patients and suggested that there is a considerable risk of lithium intoxication in patients known to severely restrict their intake, self-induce vomiting and abuse laxatives or purgatives. In a more recent study Stein and his colleagues (1982) suggested that lithium may be effective in anorexics with bulimic features.

Another drug, cyproheptadine, an antihistaminic drug, has been successfully used to promote weight gain in a variety of populations, including asthmatic children, chronically underweight adults, and adults with Irritable Bowel syndrome who were chronically underweight (Johnson et al., 1983a). In two studies with anorexics there was no difference in the amount of weight gain achieved in the drug group as opposed to a placebo (Vigersky and Loriaux, 1977; Goldberg et al., 1979). In a more recent study, however, Halmi and her colleagues suggested that cyproheptadine significantly reduced depression as rated by the Hamilton Rating Scale, compared with either amitriptyline or placebo (Halmi et al., 1983).

Until the results of further controlled trials are available, together with long-term follow-up, it may be appropriate to repeat an earlier conclusion that antidepressant treatment is not particularly indicated for anorexia nervosa but that an improvement in mood in a patient who is depressed may facilitate her general management (Szmukler, 1982).

Behaviour modification

Crisp (1977) has suggested that treatment of anorexia nervosa requires a combined behavioural and psychotherapeutic approach. Other workers too are in agreement about the importance of a behavioural approach, but the word 'behavioural' appears to mean different things to different people. Crisp (1977) views anorexia nervosa as a 'phobia' of weight gain, so that the behavioural aspect of treatment consists of exposure to the feared situation. Inpatient treatment and refeeding are behavioural in so far as the patient is thus exposed to her feared situation. Another way of exposing the patient to her feared situation is to expose her specifically through a gradual process known as 'systematic desensitisation'; but there are few reports where systematic desensitisation is used on its own (Eckert, 1983).

Many studies have described the inpatient aspect of treatment as behavioural because with weight gain patients are allowed increasingly larger numbers of privileges, such as being allowed to move about, have visitors, choose their own meals. In effect this is automatic in many programmes but in others the process is systematised to a greater or lesser degree. The use of rewards in this way to produce an increase in a desired behaviour, in this case eating, is known as operant conditioning. An alternative method is the use of negative rather than positive reinforcement, where the patient gains weight in order to avoid a negative consequence; for example, one patient had her dose of chlorpromazine reduced contingent on her gaining weight (Blinder et al., 1970).

Garfinkel and his colleagues (1973) have evaluated the effectiveness of behaviour modification by comparing the progress made in inpatient treatment, using reinforcement of weight gain, with progress made in previous hospitalisations using a variety of other treatment approaches. The seven patients studied were girls who had not responded to previous treatments and they gained on average 10.2 kilograms (22.4 lbs) in forty-two days in the behavioural condition compared to only

3.3 kg (7.3 lbs) previously. Bhanji and Thompson (1974) reported adequate weight gains in fourteen patients treated with operant conditioning, where the rewards, based on individual choice, were contingent on eating. However they noted that as some patients were still able to vomit or otherwise dispose of food, it was better to reward weight gain rather than eating.

In a sense, most programmes could be said to contain a behavioural element, as discharge is itself contingent on weight gain. In one study in fact, where extrinsic reinforcement was removed, the patient continued to gain weight (Leitenberg *et al.*, 1968). The authors investigated this further in a later study in which two patients were granted 'privileges' in return for increasing increments in weight gain. Both patients continued to gain weight when the reinforcement was removed. In a further experiment they informed the patients that the length of stay in hospital was not contingent on weight gain and under this regime the removal of positive reinforcement resulted in decreased weight gain. The authors also noted that the reinforcement was maximally effective when the patients were given feedback about how much they were eating and how much they were gaining. Moreover the larger the amount of food served, the more the patients ate (Agras *et al.*, 1974).

One of the problems of assessing the efficacy of these behaviour modification techniques in anorexia nervosa is that the treatment is often combined with other treatments, with drug therapy in particular. In a study of 'pure' behaviour modification, Halmi and her colleagues (1975) treated eight patients with positive reinforcement by social activities, increased physical activity, and visiting privileges contingent on weight gains. On average the patients gained 8.83 kg (19.4 lbs) and were in hospital for 6.25 weeks. After discharge the families of the patients were instructed to continue rewarding them for weight gains of 0.5 kg (1.1 lb) per week until they reached normal weight. The patients were followed up for up to seven months after discharge and gained on average 4.2 kg (9.2 lbs) as outpatients.

In a later paper the same authors conducted the first controlled trial of behaviour modification, where in three collaborating hospitals eighty-one anorexic patients were randomly assigned to either behaviour modification or milieu therapy and treated for five weeks. In the behaviour modification group the patients' weight gain was assessed every five days and positive reinforcement of increased social and physical activities was made contingent on weight gain. In the milieu therapy group patients could receive visitors twice a week and their post and telephone calls were not restricted. The behaviour modification group gained a little but not significantly more weight than the patients in the milieu therapy group. The authors questioned whether rewards should have been more frequent, and it is also questionable how far the negative reinforcement of being in hospital was itself a factor that linked the two treatments. In a more recent study in fact, patients on daily schedules of reinforcement gained weight more quickly than they had on a five-day fixed interval schedule (Eckert, 1983).

In a review of all controlled treatment studies of anorexia nervosa up to 1984, Agras and Kraemer have concluded that there is no difference in effectiveness between behavioural and medical therapy, although in terms of weight gain they both achieve significantly higher weights than does drug therapy. Agras and Kraemer also examined the mean length of treatment to target weight and concluded that the average of 37 days for behaviour modification was a significant improvement on the 75 days for medical therapy and 44 for drug therapy (Agras and Kraemer, 1984).

Behaviour modification has been heavily criticised by Hilde Bruch (1974a; 1983) on the basis of its not being effective in the long term, and her own experience of subsequent depression and suicide attempts in some patients. Perhaps more appropriate is the criticism that most of the so-called behavioural programmes described are not truly behavioural. We know that in order for a symptom to continue, there are factors in the environment likely to be maintaining it. In other words if something had reinforcement value for a person then taking the person out of their habitual environment and removing that reinforcement and replacing it with another will only work as long as the new programme is continued or if the newly learned habits become rewarding in themselves. Hence obsessionals treated behaviourally in hospital usually regress when they go home unless the programme has some special follow-up built into it. The only behaviour modification study that did have environmental follow-up built into it was that of Halmi and her colleagues (1975) in which the parents continued with the reinforcement at home and weight gain was in fact continued.

Clearly then something more is needed than a rigid adminis-
tration of rewards and punishments and only during inpatient
treatment. Until recently the only approach available to therapists for counselling anorexics and modifying their faulty conceptions of themselves and their bodies was psychotherapy of
one form or another.

Psychodynamic psychotherapy

Psychotherapists working in the field of anorexia nervosa have
been strongly influenced by the work of Selvini-Palazzoli and
Bruch. Both of these therapists have concluded that orthodox
psychoanalysis is inappropriate in relation to anorexia nervosa.
Selvini-Palazzoli (1978) found that translating the anorexics'
experiences into everyday language was preferable to making
'threatening' psychoanalytic interpretations, while Bruch
(1974; 1977) has commented that psychoanalysis is inappropriate for reasons connected with the nature of the disorder itself.
She has concluded that the traditional psychoanalytic setting,
in which the patient's thoughts and feelings are interpreted, is
inappropriate because of its similarity with the pattern assumed
to characterise their development, in which the patient was
constantly told by someone else what to feel and think (Bruch,
1983). Rather than nurture a feeling of ineffectiveness in such a
way Bruch suggests that the therapist must establish a rapport
with patients through allowing them to express what they
experience without necessarily explaining it or labelling it.
Patients must then be helped to express and pursue their own
needs and wants (Bruch, 1977).

Bruch recognises that the psychological problems of the
anorexic cannot truly be dealt with until the worst malnutrition
has been dealt with. She suggests that once rapport has been
established patients are able to allow themselves to be fed.
Selvini-Palazzoli (1978) similarly emphasises the notion of
rapport, saying that if patients have to be hospitalised while
under treatment they should be visited frequently in order to
maintain the feeling of trust with the therapist.

Family therapy

Both Bruch and Selvini-Palazzoli have emphasised the importance of involving the family in therapy. Bruch advocates a

setting in which the parents can acknowledge and resolve their own problems without fear of recrimination and in an atmosphere, set by the therapist, which is essentially permissive and accepting (Bruch, 1983). In her view, family therapy should be combined with individual therapy in whatever combination best suits the individual case. Treatment of the identified patient as an individual is nevertheless of prime importance in her view whatever the approach to the family.

Meanwhile, Selvini-Palazzoli has come to a rather different formulation in relation to the importance of family therapy. From 1965 onward she began to observe the transactional patterns of the families of anorexics and adopted the cybernetic view that the family is a self-regulating system based on certain rules. She concluded that members seem to be sure enough of their own communications, but that they deny the content of what other people say. No one in the family is prepared to be responsible for leadership and any decisions made are said to be for the good of someone else. The central and most serious problem is the system of alliances between members, which is based on a large number of secret rules. In addition, like Bruch, Selvini-Palazzoli sees the parents as concealing a deep disillusionment with each other which they are unable to resolve. The patient, in this system, has become the go-between. Based on these assumptions, Selvini-Palazzoli has devised a short-term form of therapy, involving the whole family and consisting of a maximum of twenty sessions.

The key to this therapy appears to be not to confront the family head-on with interpretations which would be rejected. The therapist on the contrary uses 'positive connotation'. For example, an overclose relationship between daughter and one of the parents might be redefined in terms of love and concern. A second characteristic of the therapy involves 'prescription of the symptom' where, paradoxically, the family is advised to continue behaving in a certain way. The advantages of these apparently strange tactics are that in the first place the therapist has placed herself in a position of power because she has made it impossible for the family to contradict her; and secondly by prescribing the symptom the therapist implicitly rejects it. The maintenance of neutrality is also considered extremely important. In collecting information about family interactions, the therapists use a form of circular questioning. The therapist 'cross-references' the responses from one family member to another, checking out each person's perception of the same situation, to enable the family to arrive at a new perspective on their problems (Selvini Palazzoli *et al.*, 1980).

Others have reported some success with the use of 'paradoxical intention' in the treatment of individual anorexics. For example Rosen (1980) has described a programme in which 12 eleven- to twenty-one-year-old girls abandoned their 'unacceptable' eating behaviour in response to the prescription that maladaptive behaviours should be followed all the time. Hsu and Liberman (1982) described and followed up a series of eight patients treated with a paradoxical approach. These were all patients who had failed to maintain target weight after intensive individual therapy, family therapy and re-feeding. The patients were all told, in the presence of their families, that it was better for them to keep their anorexia nervosa because previous attempts to treat them had resulted in only temporary remission of the illness. The 'benefits' of the illness were explained to the patients who were encouraged to disagree with the therapist's formulation and to continue to see him in order to explore other reasons for keeping the illness. All eight patients were seen for six one-hour sessions at weekly intervals. At follow-up of two to four years post-treatment, half the patients were at normal weight, and half had fair to good social and sexual adjustment. The authors concluded that paradoxical intention allows the therapist to ally with the ego-syntonic control mechanism in anorexia nervosa; a coalition which reduces the anorexic's need to maintain such a rigid and dangerous stance. However it may not improve social or sexual functioning and the authors advocate further psychotherapy when the patient has given up her anorectic posture.

Paradoxical intention is only one method used by family therapists. Minuchin and his colleagues, working at the same time as Selvini-Palazzoli, have devised a method of family therapy based on 'systems theory' (Minuchin *et al.*, 1978). According to this theory an individual's behaviour is seen as being both caused and causative. Like Selvini-Palazzoli its proponents see the patient very much as the product of her family, and like Selvini-Palazzoli also, they believe that it is crucial for therapy to create a change in the system. According to Minuchin and his colleagues, this implies a necessity to challenge four major family characteristics. The first of these is 'enmeshment'. This is an extreme form of proximity which leads to overinvolved family reactions and a blurring of boundaries between people and roles within the family. A second characteristic is 'overprotectiveness' – a high degree of concern for the welfare of others and restriction of the child's autonomy and competence outside the family. A third characteristic is rigidity – the family is highly committed to maintaining the status quo whatever the changing needs of the situation. A fourth characteristic is the inability of these families to resolve conflict. According to Minuchin any family might exhibit any or all of these characteristics at any one time but the important feature of 'anorexic' families is that they have no alternative way of behaving with each other, and that the symptomatic child is involved in their conflict.

Therapy, which may include hospitalisation under a behavioural (operant) regime, begins with a family lunch session during which the therapist may either 'underfocus' on the eating issue or 'overfocus' on it depending on the particular family circumstances, but will soon afterwards in subsequent sessions, move on to other issues to do with parental control in young patients, or autonomy in older adolescents. The aim of therapy is to create stress in the system, juggle with alliances, set tasks for the family, so as to take the lead in producing change in a system that is fairly rigid and unwilling to move.

Using this form of therapy, Minuchin and his colleagues have followed up fifty-three patients from one-and-a-half to seven years. Three patients dropped out of therapy but 80 per cent were followed for two or more years from the start of treatment. The authors claim 86 per cent recovery both of the anorexia and of the problems with eating behaviour. This is an extremely high success rate compared with rates claimed in other studies. Nevertheless, other therapists and research workers are ever sceptical about the efficacy of any one method taken out of context until proven through controlled trials.

In one attempt to evaluate family therapy in comparison with individual supportive therapy, Szmukler (1983) has described the problems involved in engaging families in a study where twenty-three patients were admitted to inpatient care to be followed by family therapy beginning at discharge. Eight patients defaulted, three of whom rejected the offer of follow-up care even before discharge. It is possible that if family therapy is the key, then the family needs to be engaged right from the beginning, as suggested by Minuchin and his colleagues (Minuchin *et al.*, 1978). The other factor not to be dismissed is financial. Minuchin and his colleagues make mention of the fact that their families survived treatment at a 'psychological and *financial* cost' (Minuchin *et al.*, 1978, p. 138, author's emphasis). In England, treatment is free under the National Health Service, and as will be discussed in relation to the treatment of obesity, this may be yet another crucial factor to be considered in relation to the success or otherwise of treatment.

Behavioural therapy aimed at self-control and attitude change

Current thinking in behaviour therapy has come a long way from the time when most therapies were based on Pavlovian conditioning, or operant conditioning with its implication that the patient's responses to his environment can be altered in a way analogous to the pigeon's learning to peck in order to receive food that is thrown down a chute. Current formulations take into account the notion that the person can himself be taught to control his own environment, to control the stimuli that cue him to behave in certain ways and hence to achieve control over his own behaviour. In relation to the treatment of anorexia nervosa, behaviour therapy still has some way to go in this direction but there are a few signs that behaviourally oriented therapists are attempting like Bruch, though in a different way, to give the power back to the anorexic herself. For example, in one single case study a bulimic anorexic patient was encouraged to bring desired food to her sessions. After eating part of the food she was exposed to the rest for thirty minutes and was taught to do the same herself at home (Smith and Medlik, 1983). Others have used a combination of contingency contracting and other techniques such as self-monitoring (recording all food eaten and problems which arise) and graded exposure to high salience food situations (Cinciprini *et al.*, 1983). These approaches apply best of course to anorexics who binge-eat, as they focus on learning control in the face of 'prohibited' food rather than on learning to eat more.

Another promising approach, however, which may have applications for both restricting and bulimic anorexics, is the use of cognitive behavioural psychotherapy. Garner and Bemis (1982) and Fairburn (1984) have expressed optimism about the utility of this approach. The therapy is one which is designed not just to change behaviour but to change the patient's underlying assumptions and misconceptions. One form of cognitive therapy was developed by Beck and his colleagues (1976) for the treatment of depression, and in controlled trials has compared favourably with drug treatment even for very depressed patients.

Cognitive therapy, according to Beck, is an 'active, directive, time-limited, structured approach' (Beck, 1976, p. 3). It is based on the underlying rationale that the patient's feelings and behaviour are determined by the way in which he structures the world, and the therapy itself consists of setting up hypotheses on the basis of the patient's attitudes and experiences and testing them systematically. For example, if the patient believes he is incapable of a task, the therapist and he together might draw up a checklist or graph which he can use to record how much success he actually has in carrying out the task. The emphasis is on 'collaborative empiricism' in which both therapist and client are active in a joint venture.

In some respects there are similarities with Bruch's formulations. For example she talks of therapy as representing an attempt 'to repair the conceptual defects and distortions' (Bruch, 1983) and of the therapist as 'engaging the patient as a *collaborator*' (author's emphasis). Cognitive therapy differs from Bruch's work in that it is not based on the same theory of aetiology. It takes account of the notion that the way in which the disorder has developed may be very different from one individual to the next. Another major difference is that as well as providing feedback, cognitive behavioural therapy structures the experience of the patient and provides new strategies for use in solving problems relating to the disorder and the patient's misconceptions. Theoretically also it should be possible to standardise techniques and thus allow for the therapy to be replicated and its effects tested empirically (Garner and Bemis, 1982).

Garner and Bemis (1982) hold that the Socratic dialogue embodied in cognitive therapy lends itself well to therapy with patients who typically function at a level of constant self-examination and who have difficulty in describing 'true feelings'. They suggest that therapy includes a didactic element in which the patient is given information about the effects of starvation. They suggest that the techniques of cognitive therapy with its emphasis on fostering a sound therapeutic relationship and its use of the experimental model, provide a rational approach to the anorexic who typically does not wish to change and is wary of therapists who may be perceived as agents of coercion. In a paper in which they describe in detail their modification of Beck's cognitive therapy techniques, they have described the reasoning errors which they have observed most frequently in anorexic patients (Garner and Bemis, 1982). These are: dichotomous or all-or-none reasoning; personalisation and self-reference – for example the idea that other people will notice that the patient is too fat, or the interpretation of neutral events, looks or glances, as signs of rejection or criticism; superstitious thinking – whereby the patient has the magical belief in cause-effect relationships between unrelated events, such as belief that laxative abuse or vomiting absolves her of guilt from overeating. Underlying these reasoning errors are basic 'assumptions' from which many of the person's attitudes are derived. A common assumption, experienced by depressives, anorexics and patients with many other neurotic disorders alike, is that it is of crucial importance to be liked by everyone. Garner and Bemis (1982) have added others, such as 'fat is intrinsically bad' and 'perfect performance is necessary for self-fulfillment'.

Like Beck (1976) both Garner and Bemis (1982) emphasise the importance of not simply challenging the patient about these assumptions. The goal of the therapy is in the first place to elicit them from the patient in such a way that she herself recognises them, and secondly to work with her to gather evidence in support of or against them; to test out the assumptions and to consider how far they apply in reality and how they might be modified.

More recently Cooper and Fairburn (1984) have reported some preliminary evaluation of a form of cognitive therapy with five patients treated by them. The treatment was in two phases. In the first phase the patients were given information about the effects of starvation and encouraged to increase their eating with the promise that they would be helped to maintain control. They were given instructions about the appropriate foods to eat in order to promote weight gain. The second phase was begun only after significant weight gain. In this phase emphasis was on dealing with loss of control (Fairburn, 1981). The patients were taught to monitor their eating behaviour and to recognise events and moods concomitant with disordered eating. In order to deal with these the patients were taught problem-solving techniques, a form of cognitive restructuring, similar to the approach of Goldfried and Goldfried (1975). Like Garner and Bemis's patients they were also encouraged to identify and replace irrational thoughts. The authors imply that their method is rather more didactic than that described by Garner and Bemis. They cite Meichenbaum (1977) whose training procedure is more active than that of Beck. Patients are taught to monitor irrational internal dialogues and the therapist then models more adaptive dialogues which the patient is encouraged to copy and learn. In Beck's therapy the alternative strategies come from the patient himself as a result of the dialogue with the therapist in which negative thoughts and assumptions are questioned and more positive thoughts are elicited from the patient's replies.

In addition to the cognitive strategies, Fairburn used other behavioural strategies, in particular graded exposure to previously 'banned' foods (Fairburn, 1981).

Using this approach Cooper and Fairburn claimed some success at one-year follow-up with the patients in their group who suffered from bulimia. The restricting patients, however, did not benefit at all from the treatment. These latter patients were also the thinnest of the group, at less than 65 per cent of matched population mean weight. It is possible that patients who have reached a high level of starvation are less amenable to any kind of psychological intervention until their weight has been increased. Alternatively it may be that as Fairburn and Cooper have suggested, the therapy techniques devised by them are more specific to patients with disordered eating habits than to patients who rely on restriction alone.

Cognitive therapy has a certain rational appeal for the treatment of anorexia nervosa, in particular for engaging a reluctant patient in therapy. It combines the practical behavioural with Bruch's notion of 'collaboration' and promises a solution for the

146

dilemma of long-term control. It remains to be seen, however, how far the newer approaches embodied in conjoint family therapy and individual cognitive therapy respectively will come up to the expectations of their proponents and improve the long-term social and emotional prospects of a severely disabled group.

11 Treatment of obesity

Overweight carries with it increased mortality and morbidity. Overweight people are at increased risk compared with other people for many diseases including coronary artery disease, high blood pressure, diabetes mellitus and gall bladder disease (Royal College of Physicians, 1983; Simopoulos, 1985).

In the light of these risks, the crusade against obesity has in the past twenty to thirty years gone from strength to strength. Medical doctors have been joined in battle by armies of surgeons, nutritionists, psychologists and commercial slimming clubs in a battle which, in view of the increasing weights of people in the Western world, is a battle lost.

Most treatments of obesity have focussed on the assumed overeating of the obese person. Hence their aim is usually to reduce appetite, to prevent large amounts of food being absorbed, to instruct the patient in eating less or to reduce the availability of food.

Methods used for weight loss depend to some extent on the degree of overweight of the obese patient. The need for a person with a W/H^2 index of over 40, or 100 per cent overweight is more urgent than for a moderately obese person whose W/H^2 is 25 to 30. (Garrow, 1981). It is in relation to these people that the battle for a medical treatment other than diet alone has been fought most seriously.

Medical treatment

Surgical procedures

Twenty-one different surgical procedures have been developed for the treatment of obesity (Kral, 1983). Most surgeons have agreed that the criterion for considering a patient for surgical

148

treatment is 100 per cent overweight, or that the patient has at least 45 kilograms to lose. Younger patients who have much to gain by the improvement resulting from weight loss, and patients who it can be predicted will comply with the demands of the long-term follow-up necessitated by treatment, are those normally chosen.

Jejunoileal bypass was developed in the mid-1950s. There have been several different versions of this operation which in effect creates a loop in the intestine with the aim of decreasing the amount of food which can be digested or absorbed. In fact the operation results in reduced food intake, both in animals and man.

Another operative procedure is the gastric bypass. There is a variety of types, all having the effect mainly of allowing the patient to eat less through reducing the size of the stomach. This operation also carries certain complications, for example perforations in the upper or lower stomach which can cause death (Mason *et al.*, 1980). Side-effects in the post-operative period include post-prandial vomiting and distension owing to intake in excess of pouch size (Buchwald, 1980). The gastric bypass operation also has its side-effects including unremitting nausea and vomiting and failure to lose weight. Moreover the gastric bypass procedure can be out-eaten by every patient through continuous snacking (Buchwald, 1980). Patients may lose only a minimal amount of weight, may lose no weight at all, or even gain weight. Two to 5 per cent of the bypasses have to be revised or taken down.

Champions of these operative procedures claim that most patients are happy with the results, despite the sometimes dangerous risks taken and the discomfort associated with the after-effects of surgery and that associated with eating, possibly into the long-term. On the other hand there arises the question of whether people should be subjected to these procedures at all, considering the risks and discomfort. Patients who demand surgery are fairly desperate people. They have tried and failed many times to lose weight through dieting. This being so, it is very difficult to predict who will, and who will not, comply with medical advice after the operation so as to achieve the best outcome. Wooley, Wooley and Dyrenforth (1980) have raised the question of whether informed consent prior to operation is as comprehensive as it could be. They hold that the only difference between operative procedures and diet is that the former guarantees compliance. Yet the patients should be given the opportunity to experience other methods, together with the opportunity to consider the meaning of overweight and the necessity of becoming thinner.

Jaw-wiring

A less intrusive physical means of reducing weight is jaw-wiring. This procedure is self-explanatory. The patient literally has his or her mouth 'locked' so that he or she is unable to eat. The purpose of this is to make it easier for the patient to keep to a diet restricted to milk which contains most of the nutrients needed. There is of course always a way around the wires just as there is round any diet. Normal food can be liquidised or small items of food pushed through the necessary gaps between the wires. However the intention of the wiring is not to make this impossible, but to reduce the availability of food (Garrow, 1981). Another serious problem is the rate at which patients often regain their weight once the wires have been removed. Success with a period of jaw-wiring was previously used by Garrow as a prerequisite for gastric bypass, as this was thought to give some indication of the patient's level of compliance. More recently, however, he has preferred the less risky method of maintaining weight loss after jaw-wiring by use of the waist cord (Garrow and Gardiner, 1981). Patients who ask to have their jaws wired are contracted also to having a cord fixed round their waists when they have reached goal weight. The cord is there as a reminder, like tight clothes, if the patient puts on weight, and cannot be removed or loosened except by the physician. Using this technique, Garrow and Gardiner have claimed success in maintaining weight by four patients whose jaws had been wired compared with others who had had their jaws wired without subsequent waist-cord follow-up. One of the problems with this kind of treatment is that outcome in part depends on the relationship of the patients with their physician and linked with this the motivation to keep the waist cord on. Many patients undergo severe discomfort around the waist rather than cut the cord and allow themselves to regain their lost weight (Garrow, personal communication). Thus many patients manage to control their weight, but not necessarily their eating habits. If the waist cord is effective, it is a cheap and probably harmless means of losing or maintaining weight. It remains to be seen whether its effectiveness will be demonstrated more widely, and what is its method of action. The question arises as to whether patients learn to maintain their weight by modifying their eating habits or by keeping to a well balanced diet; or whether they become at worst like bulimics who are able to maintain their weight only through alternate bingeing and starving or at best like some people in behavioural programmes who take nutritionally unsound diets (see page 160).

Drug treatment

Drugs used have been mainly appetite depressant, and include amphetamine, phentermine, diethylproprion, mazindol, and fenfluramine. [Common side-effects which have been reported in all to a varying degree have been insomnia, nervousness, dry mouth, lethargy and constipation] (Munro and Ford, 1982). There is also a small potential for abuse not only with amphetamine but also with mazindol, fenfluramine, phentermine, and diethylproprion, in that patients may become psychologically dependent on their stimulant effect (Royal College of Physicians, 1983). In controlled double-blind trials, patients given anorectic drugs have lost more weight than those on placebo. However, [the drugs do not modify eating habits, and losses are not maintained long-term] (Munro, 1979). There is of course the additional problem of compliance. In a study in which 48 patients had to collect their monthly drug ration from the hospital pharmacy, only 4 women and 1 man collected more than 6 prescriptions (Gilbert and Garrow, 1983), and not all pills collected were actually taken.

Psychodynamic treatment for obese people

Psychodynamic therapy involves treatment of the personal problems of the dieter. Hilde Bruch (1974) has pointed out that it is appropriate only for those overweight people who are psychiatrically disturbed or depressed. The therapy does not make reducing itself any easier, but theoretically increased self-knowledge enables the individual to tolerate better the problems of dieting. According to Bruch (1974), obese people are unresponsive to traditional psychoanalysis as are anorexics, and the therapy must be tailored to meet their individual problems. It is not usually appropriate to generalise about the nature of this kind of therapy; however Bruch does also point out that the patient needs to be encouraged away from intense emotional involvement with her parents and encouraged towards independence.

The approach is the antithesis of a purely medical approach whereby massively overweight people who claim that their problems would be over if only they could have an operation, their jaws wired, a magic pill, are treated by a direct attack on the weight itself. A psychodynamic approach rests on the assumption that there are some overweight people for whom stuffing and starving or maintaining a high weight serves a purpose in relation to that person's psychological functioning. If this is the case then a direct attack on the weight is both senseless and damaging. The 'cure' lies in the direction of increased understanding of self, and of the reasons for overeating; and acceptance if necessary of a higher than normal weight.

A major criticism of this kind of approach is that it does not lend itself, as does medical treatment, to measurement of outcome. The outcome measure most usually applied is, of course, weight itself, but in relation to psychotherapy a good outcome might, or might not, be accompanied by weight loss. Thus it cannot be compared as a treatment with other therapies for overweight, and it becomes largely a question of belief. Critics may dismiss it out of hand, whereas others may agree with the approach but are in the uncomfortable position of being unable to substantiate their belief. The answer is in finding more appropriate measures than weight alone; for example of self-esteem, or satisfaction with body size.

One attempt has been made to assess the effects of psychoanalysis on obesity. This is a four-year follow-up of information about 84 obese and 63 non-obese patients (Rand and Stunkard, 1978, 1983). One hundred and four psychoanalysts were asked to provide questionnaire information on their obese patients and on non-obese patients matched for age, sex and race. Seventy-two analysts replied, and the survey was repeated at eighteen months and four years. The data obtained was the subjective judgment of the analyst, and over-weight was defined as 'somebody clearly looking fat who is 20 per cent or more overweight'. The first survey reported on a median duration of 33 months of treatment, and according to the analysts weight loss in the obese patients averaged 4.5kg. At eighteen-months follow-up it had increased to an average of 9.5kg and at 4 years to 11.6kg. The questionnaire also reported on 'body image disparagement'. The analysts reported a decrease in this problem over the time period of the surveys, a decrease not associated with degree of weight loss, however. Patients rated improved by their analysts also lost significantly more weight than those rated unimproved. The authors suggest that the study presents some evidence that treatment by psychoanalysis may be helpful in both reducing weight and maintaining losses in the long term. The chief criticism of this kind of study of course is the subjective nature of the reports – definition of overweight depended on a subjective decision by the analyst, and all weight losses were reports by the analysts of self-reports by the patients. Moreover, the patients themselves were a highly selected group of upper middle-class people, who could afford the lengthy treatment involved. Criticisms aside, it is feasible that long-term psychological therapy is helpful for some people in achieving and maintaining weight loss. The problem remains, however, of whether and to what extent improvements might be achieved for the majority of overweight people at a lesser cost both financially and in terms of time.

Hypnosis

A treatment which many people, in particular self-confessed overeaters, ask about is hypnosis. Hypnosis has the popular image of a kind of magic; something that will cast a spell over the person who will no longer need to eat to excess and who will have a newfound 'willpower'.

Many claims are made for the effects of hypnosis, particularly in the advertisements in the personal columns of magazines and newspapers. However, the literature relating to hypnotherapy for weight reduction consists mainly of anecdotal reports and uncontrolled studies of selected cases. Mott and Roberts (1979) have reviewed the literature and have noted that techniques vary from one study to another. Many people report

153

success, but often degree of overweight is not given, or there is no follow-up, so that it is impossible to assess the efficacy of hypnotherapy itself *vis-à-vis* other forms of treatment or to assess which aspects in particular are effective. Wadden and Flaxman (1981) compared hypnosis with behaviour therapy in a seven-week study of mildly overweight women and concluded that subjects in all conditions did equally well. Others have used hypnosis as an adjunct to behaviour therapy with some success (Ringrose, 1979; Bolocofsky *et al.*, 1985). It remains to be seen how far this success may be attributable to a specific aspect of hypnotic procedures, or to procedures which in fact are very similar to those of behaviour therapy itself.

Behaviour therapy

Behaviour therapy is the most widely used formal treatment for obesity today, at least in the United States (Foreyt and Kondo, 1984). Behaviour therapy is a term which covers a wide variety of treatment approaches.

One behavioural approach in which many patients and professionals alike express interest is aversive conditioning. Because of its use in relation to other addictive and habit disorders, this approach has some popular appeal. However, the results of studies in which aversive stimuli such as electric shocks are paired with food, or in which food images are paired with aversive scenes, are equivocal (Foreyt and Kennedy, 1971; Foreyt and Hagen, 1973). At best it may be possible to reduce the palatability of a favourite food in the short term through pairing with an aversive stimulus (Abramson and Jones, 1981) but there is no evidence that aversive conditioning can produce long-term weight loss. This is not surprising in view of the fact that in general positive reinforcement is more effective than punishment as a means of fostering behavioural change. However, it is an important point to make, as obese people are prone to being self-punitive, guilty about their condition, and may easily fall prey to and allow themselves to be treated by systems containing a punitive element. Many trudge weekly or monthly to visit their general practitioners, dietitians, or hospital outpatient clinics, only to be chastised for non-compliance with advice to lose weight. It is important for health professionals to avoid the temptation to be drawn into this kind of pattern, which does neither the patient nor the therapist any good.

Stuart's study entitled 'The behavioural control of overeating' became the forerunner to a vast literature on the use of behavioural methods in the treatment of obesity (Stuart, 1967). The study was based on the hypothesis of Ferster, Nurnberger and Levitt (1962) that obese people eat in response to a variety of external cues and in a style which causes them to overeat. Stuart (1967) described in detail the results of treatment of 8 subjects followed up over 16 to 41 sessions in one year. Three subjects lost more than 18 kg, and 6 more than 13.75kg. Supported also by the Schachterian hypothesis of 'externality' (see Chapter 7), Stuart and Davis expanded the methods into a programme which was to become the basis of some 200 further studies on the behavioural treatment of obesity. The programme included monitoring intake, modifying cues that signal 'inappropriate eating', modifying the act of eating itself, increasing exercise, and self-reward for more appropriate behaviour (Stuart and Davis, 1972). Self-monitoring means keeping a written record of everything eaten and of the circumstances in which it was eaten – the time of day, where, who with, and also of what was happening prior to eating, or of what kind of mood the person was in. The idea of the record is that dieters should become more aware of inappropriate eating habits, such as eating when bored, or eating in response to seeing food rather than in response to 'hunger'. Eliminating the cues that signal inappropriate eating includes controlling the environment in which the person eats, for example changing habits such as snacking while watching TV or reading. Temptation to eat is reduced by shopping only from a list, and avoiding unnecessary contact with high calorie food by keeping favourite snacks out of reach, asking family members to prepare their own snacks, or throwing leftovers away rather than attempting to save them. Modifying the act of eating itself is achieved by eating more slowly, perhaps even counting mouthfuls per minute, and using utensils at all times to reduce the possibility of uncontrolled snacking. Programme behaviours are introduced sometimes all together at the same time, and sometimes in stages, in consecutive sessions. Clients are taught how to select long- and short-term rewards which they gain through achievement of target behaviours. They are also encouraged to reward themselves for taking increasing amounts of exercise, such as walking an extra bus stop, parking their car further away from their place of work, or playing a sport.

Several researchers have subjected these methods, or aspects of the methods, to increasingly stringent scrutiny in an attempt to replicate Stuart's excellent results. In 1972, in a paper entitled 'New therapies for the eating disorders' Stunkard claimed that 'both greater weight loss during treatment and superior maintenance of weight loss after treatment indicate that behaviour modification is more effective than previous methods of treatment for obesity' (Stunkard, 1972). Few people, however, have matched Stuart's results and opinion as to the efficacy of behaviour therapy changes from year to year and from one reviewer to the next. In 1979 Stunkard himself was disappointed to conclude that 'clinically important weight losses achieved by behavioural treatments for obesity are not well maintained' (Stunkard and Penick, 1979). How effective then is behaviour therapy, and how does it compare with other treatments for obesity?

Does behaviour therapy work?

The first person to address the question of efficacy since Stuart's original study was Harris (1969). He treated mildly overweight college students in an eight-week behavioural programme. They lost an average of 4.75kg compared to a no-treatment control group who gained 1.5kg. Treated subjects, moreover, continued to lose a further 0.9kg during four months' follow-up. Wollersheim (1970) subsequently addressed the question of whether the behavioural programme was itself responsible for the weight loss rather than other features of treatment. She assigned seventy-nine overweight college students to one of four experimental conditions: social pressure, non-specific therapy, focal therapy based on learning principles, and a no-treatment waiting list control. At both post-treatment and eight-week follow-up, the focal group lost more weight. However, while this study controlled for the subjects' expectations of therapy, it could be open to criticism on the grounds of experimenter bias. A study by Penick and his colleagues (1971) attempted to control for this. The first author himself ran a conventional therapy group with seventeen patients, while behaviour therapy groups for fifteen patients were run by inexperienced therapists. Once more the results favoured the behavioural treatment, although intersubject variability suggested a specific effect. The study was of interest also because it achieved success with a patient group rather than the often-used moderately overweight student group; and in that treatment was effective in the hands of inexperienced therapists. Subsequent studies have used non-professionals or individuals not primarily trained as psychological therapists with some success (Stunkard and Brownell, 1980; Brownell *et al.*, 1985). Clearly this is an advantage for behaviour therapy in relation to the cost of treatment. Nevertheless weight losses achieved may vary between therapists (Beneke and Paulsen, 1979; Kirschenbaum *et al.*, 1985); and therapists do still need to be highly trained as there is some evidence that weight losses correlate with their experience (Levitz and Stunkard, 1974; Jeffery *et al.*, 1978; Koch and Gromus, 1983).

Related to the question of the training of the therapist is that of whether the therapist is needed at all. Many programmes produce a manual for patients as part of the therapy programme and several studies have looked at the use of bibliotherapy as an adjunct to or as an alternative to the therapist. For example Hagen (1974) divided 90 students into three treatment groups: group therapy, bibliotherapy, and group therapy with bibliotherapy. The treatments were equally effective but subjects who attended the groups felt that they had been more helped than did those in the manual-alone condition. Others have conducted similar experiments and concluded that bibliotherapy or therapy by mail is as effective as high contact (Bellack, Schwartz and Rozensky, 1974; Jeffery *et al.*, 1982). The evidence is confusing, however, as in other studies subjects are reported to have lost more weight in the short term with programmed texts and minimal contact with therapists than with high-contact conditions (Hanson *et al.*, 1976; Brownell *et al.*, 1978). In yet other studies moderately overweight women were less likely to drop out of treatment if they met their therapists more often (Brownell *et al.*, 1985) and to lose more weight on a course of ten sessions with a therapist than on a correspondence course of ten sessions with similar content (Baanders-Van Halewijn *et al.*, 1984).

The discrepancies between findings in the studies which

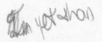

investigate the effects of varying degrees of therapist contact may of course relate to characteristics of the clients treated or to other components of the treatment package itself. Other studies have focussed on the efficacy of specific components of behaviour therapy itself. For example, self-monitoring is an important though not exclusively effective component of treatment (Romanczyk, 1974; Romanczyk et al., 1973). On the whole clients do better when they reward themselves for habit change than for weight loss (Wilson and Brownell 1980).

In terms of weight loss few studies have been as effective as Stuart's (1967) original study. Jeffery, Wing and Stunkard (1978) in a review of the results from 21 behavioural studies found an average weight loss of 5.2kg during treatment, which other reviewers have agreed holds stable across all treatments. This is a statistically but usually not clinically significant amount of weight. Stuart (1980) has himself criticised the majority of behavioural programmes for obesity on several counts. For example he points out that the usual eight- to twelve-week programme offered is an incomplete service, as few people, losing at 0.5kg to 1 kg per week, can reach goal weight in that time. Few researchers specify prescriptions for food intake and energy expenditure requirements so that people in behavioural weight loss programmes may be losing weight on inappropriate diets. Not enough programmes carry out a thorough behavioural and functional analysis so as to deal with individual urges to eat rather than merely rewarding clients for specific behavioural changes; and few programmes include continuous monitoring of clients' degree of compliance.

These considerations are particularly important considering that the long-term effects of behaviour therapy are somewhat mixed. Only about 10 per cent of studies have reported on follow-up of ten months or more. Of these, perhaps one third show a loss at follow-up compared to the post-treatment measure. In most the figures indicate that subjects have on average begun to regain weight although there is still a net loss compared to pretreatment. To some extent averaged results are misleading as there is wide variability between individual subjects. Stunkard and Penick (1979) have reported that subjects who lost weight in their treatment studies did not necessarily continue to do so afterwards, while others who failed to lose during treatment tended to lose during follow-up. During their five-year follow-up this relationship continued but weight was gradually regained. Other studies with follow-up of more than one year have shown similar trends back to pre-treatment weights (Gotestam, 1979; O'Neil *et al.*, 1980; Graham *et al.*, 1983). Nevertheless, some subjects do continue to lose weight (Brightwell *et al.*, 1980), or at least to maintain significant net losses up to six years after treatment (Jordan *et al.*, 1985).

Improving long-term maintenance in behaviour therapy

There has been a series of attempts at improving follow-up results in behaviour therapy, using booster sessions. These are essentially follow-up sessions which repeat the message of behavioural sessions to date. Subjects who attend booster sessions maintain their losses in the short term, as long as they are still in treatment but only if they continue with the same therapist. Long-term follow-up results using this technique are not particularly promising, however (Hall *et al.*, 1975; Ashby and Wilson, 1977; Kingsley and Wilson, 1977). More recently, several writers have attempted to vary the type of long-term follow-up offered to ascertain what if any strategies might improve long-term maintenance. For example, Wing and his colleagues divided clients who had completed a behavioural weight control programme into one of three conditions: where all clients were weighed weekly but attended a follow-up group under three different contingencies: noncontingent on weight loss, contingent on continued weight loss, or contingent only on weight gain. However the contingencies had no effect on long-term attendance or weight loss (Wing *et al.*, 1984). There is, however, some evidence that whereas booster sessions on their own are not particularly helpful, strategies aimed at teaching clients how to help themselves may result in better maintenance. Examples of these are: learning how to form peer groups for mutual support; and receiving intensive group or individual training in problem-solving techniques after initial treatment or during initial treatment followed by faded mail or telephone contact with the therapist. These strategies all appear to compare favourably with the use of booster sessions or non-specific follow-up sessions in the maintenance of weight loss after treatment (Perri *et al.*, 1984, 1984a; Jeffery *et al.*, 1984; Björvell and Rössner, 1985).

TREATMENT OF THE EATING DISORDERS

Nevertheless there is a risk in attaching too much importance to the long-term effects of therapy. Many people go on to join other programmes which may or may not include a behavioural element (Graham *et al.*, 1983). As important therefore is how well behaviour therapy stands up to comparison with other treatments.

The efficacy of behaviour therapy in comparison with other treatments for obesity

The crucial test of behaviour therapy as well as its efficacy in both the short and the long term is, of course, its power as a treatment in comparison with other available treatments. Over-all, the drop-out rate from therapy is in general lower at between 0 and 26 per cent than in traditional medical treatment where it may be as high as 80 per cent (Wilson and Brownell, 1980).

Most earlier comparisons with other therapies have been with non-focal therapies, and results are in favour of behaviour therapy although not always in the long term. The few studies that have compared behavioural with diet-alone treatments have come out heavily in favour of the behavioural. This is true for treatment of adults (Harmatz and Lapuc, 1968; Levitz and Stunkard, 1974; Gormally and Rardin, 1981) and for children (Epstein *et al.*, 1980). In one study comparing nutrition education with behavioural counselling the two groups did equally well during treatment; but the people in the behavioural condition followed nutritionally unsound diets, although they maintained their losses better in the long term (Gormally and Rardin, 1981). More recently Kirschenbaum and his colleagues (1985) have compared behavioural therapies with intensive non-specific therapies in which subjects were asked to execute programme behaviours just as time-consuming as those in the behavioural treatment. The subjects in the non-specific therapies did as well even at two-year follow-up as did those in the behavioural groups, but they did report changes in eating behaviour. The authors suggested that people may have become more sophisticated about methods of losing weight and that the importance of group pressure cannot be underestimated.

There have been several attempts to compare the effects of

160

drugs with behavioural treatment. Dahms and his colleagues (1978) compared behaviour therapy with two drugs and a placebo in 120 outpatients. There were no differences in the results but the study was characterised by a 75 per cent attrition rate. In our own controlled outpatient study comparing the effects of drug therapy with behaviour therapy the drop-out rate was similar to that described by Dahms *et al*. and there was no difference between weight losses in the drug and behavioural conditions at one year (Gilbert and Garrow, 1983). In contrast, Stunkard and his colleagues, with a more highly selected group of patients, found superior in-treatment results with fenflur-amine and with a combination treatment compared to be-haviour therapy alone (Stunkard *et al*., 1980). Results of a study by Abramson and his colleagues (1980) are comparable with those of Stunkard and his colleagues for the first twelve weeks of treatment, with patients in a combined therapy group losing more weight than patients in a behaviour therapy plus placebo group. Similar results are also claimed in combination treatment studies by Brightwell and Naylor (1979) and Bigelow and his colleagues (1980). Stunkard and his colleagues, how-ever, were the first to report on follow-up of the behavioural versus drug versus combination treatments. One-year follow-up of all the patients who completed treatment showed a reversal of the treatment effects, in that behaviour therapy patients gained significantly less of the lost weight than the pharmacotherapy and combined therapy patients.

Hence in the short term, behavioural and drug therapies may be equally effective at producing weight loss, but where more subjects remain in treatment drug therapy may produce greater losses. This does not appear to hold true in the long term where behaviour therapy alone is more resistant to relapse. Patients given some self-help skills may be able to use these for longer compared with patients for whom therapy has been externally imposed.

Behaviour therapy in combination with other therapies for obesity

In view of the good short-term effects of several therapies, and the apparent success of behavioural techniques in improving maintenance, many researchers have developed combination treatments. Thus, for example, in one uncontrolled study Miller and Sims provided an intensive four-week programme combining behaviour therapy with diet, nutritional education, medical and health education and exercise (Miller and Sims, 1981). Mean weight loss one year after treatment was 13.2 kilograms, double that of many other programmes. Success with low-calorie diet combined with behavioural techniques has also been claimed in other follow-up studies, which have reported losses of up to 20 or 30 kilograms in six months.

Stifler (1983), using a protein-sparing modified fast in combination with behavioural techniques, claimed losses of on average 29 kg. over six and a half months, with 74 per cent of patients maintaining 80 per cent of their losses five months later. Similarly, Wadden and his colleagues (1984) treated seventeen women, all at least 50 per cent overweight, with a combined programme. In six months the women had lost on average 20.5 kilograms and one year later the twelve women who were traced still weighed on average 19.8 kilograms less than they had at the beginning of the programme.

As a result of the short-term success of drug therapy and the longer-term maintenance effects of behaviour therapy in a previous study (Stunkard et al., 1980), Craighead (1984) investigated the use of behaviour therapy and drug therapy in combination. Subjects received behaviour therapy, or medication, or combined therapy, for sixteen weeks. The combined therapy consisted of behaviour therapy with medication being added either in the first eight weeks or in the last eight weeks of treatment. Weight loss was increased more in the short term by adding pharmacotherapy in the last phase of treatment rather than in the first phase. Medication was also particularly helpful in speeding up weight loss in those who had not responded to behaviour therapy, but on long-term follow-up the differences were no longer significant.

Behaviour therapy has also been used successfully in combination with exercise programmes (Dahlkoetter et al., 1979; Epstein et al., 1984; Miller and Sims, 1981). It is not clear as yet how far exercise adds to the degree of actual weight lost and how far it has its effect through enhancing maintenance.

What behaviour change leads to weight loss?

Response to behaviour therapy is itself extremely varied. This is not entirely surprising if we take into account the notion that the assumptions on which it is based may to some extent be unfounded. We now know that not all overweight people overeat, are more responsive to external cues, or have a different eating style from people of normal weight (see Chapter 7). There is no reason therefore to suppose that all fat people might necessarily lose weight as a result of such technical tricks as eating more slowly, eating only in one place or with the same utensils. Besides, even if these behaviours are the most appropriate, it is difficult to ascertain how far doing them actually results in weight loss, considering that in the first place two people behaving in the same way could well lose at different rates, and in the second place they may not do as they have been advised. Brownell and Stunkard (1978) have argued that the link between compliance with programmes and weight loss is non-existent. To some extent this may relate to the nature of the measures used, and the most specific measures may not always be the most appropriate.

Self-reports of increased exercise have been associated with success both in losing and in maintaining weight losses in several studies (Miller and Sims, 1981; Katahn *et al.*, 1982; and Colvin and Olsen, 1983). Where food-related behaviours are concerned, however, the associations are less clear-cut. Successful dieters have claimed more consistent use of self-monitoring than have unsuccessful dieters (Bellack, Schwartz and Rozensky, 1974; Colvin and Olson, 1983). Sandifer and Buchanan (1983) reported finding significant correlations between programme behaviours such as eating only in a designated food area, refraining from other activities during meals and in particular pausing between mouthfuls. However Stalonas and his colleagues (1978) who also had subjects continuously monitoring habit change and therapists rating the changes, found that of several measures, only 'uncontrolled eating' was significantly correlated with weight change. Jeffery, Vender and Wing found weight reduction to be correlated with only 5 out of 20 measures. Only the use of self-monitoring and situational restriction correlated significantly with weight reduction (Jeffery, Vender and Wing, 1978). Change in self-reported thoughts about food on the other hand was the best predictor of weight reduction. Other studies have been similarly non-specific in their findings. For example, Heckerman and Prochaska (1976) reported retrospectively a correlation between weight reduction and the extent to which subjects reported understanding and execution of homework assignments. Possibly the development of a belief in newfound control of overeating is as important as the execution of the behaviours themselves. Both Hagen (1974) and Wollersheim (1970) using Wollersheim's Eating Patterns Questionnaire, found correlations between weight loss and changes in self-reports of uncontrolled eating, eating in isolation, and eating between meals. These findings are consistent with those of more recent studies in which patients who report increasing success in the use of problem-solving (Black and Scherba, 1983) and cognitive restructuring techniques (Miller and Sims, 1981) are among those most successful at losing weight.

Thus there is not necessarily a direct relationship between eating habit change and weight loss. It has been estimated that the eating habits measured in behavioural programmes may account for only about 20 per cent of the variance in weight loss (Stalonas and Kirschenbaum, 1985). A factor which may be more important is the degree to which subjects in behavioural weight control studies are able to make overall changes. This does not imply that compliance with specific programme behaviours is unimportant. On the contrary, it supports the notion that in order to lose the same amount of weight, subjects of differing metabolic rate and with differing life-styles may need to make eating habit changes of differing degree.

The crucial test of a behavioural weight control programme, then, may be how far it enables subjects to learn the use of behavioural techniques with which they can tackle their own specific problems in relation both to losing weight and to avoiding relapse.

Using behavioural methods to increase compliance with therapy

While obese people do not necessarily eat more than or in a different way from people of normal weight, clearly those who are able to make the biggest changes in their life-style are most likely to lose weight and to maintain their losses. Behavioural change is nevertheless extremely difficult for most people and the more complex the behaviour change required of patients the less likely they are to comply with treatment in general (Haynes, 1976). To lose weight requires that patients comply with many new rules, and continue to do so for some considerable time.

One important measure of compliance is the level of attrition. The number of people who drop out of treatment is to some extent unknown. In a review of twenty-one studies of outpatient treatment Wing and Jeffery (1979) noted that 19 per cent of studies reviewed did not mention drop-outs at all. Where reported, drop-out appeared similar across behavioural, anorectic drug and diet studies. This finding is somewhat at variance with the conclusion of Wilson and Brownell (1980) that attrition in controlled behavioural studies is lower than in relation to other treatments. Probably it is reasonable to conclude that low drop-out rates, where they occur, do so most frequently in relation to the behavioural studies. The problem then is to ascertain what factors are responsible for the large degree of variability. Drop-out would have little importance if we had evidence that people who drop out are as likely to lose weight as people who stay in treatment. Most studies do not follow drop-outs, but in our own study of 115 outpatients we did succeed in tracing 85 per cent of people one year after enrolment, and were able to ascertain that weight loss at one year was significantly related to attendance at the clinic (Gilbert and Garrow, 1983).

Similarly in a study of behaviour therapy, attendance was related both to short and long-term success (Jeffery *et al.*, 1984). In our own study there was no evidence that longer attendance resulted in weight loss as a result of increased exposure to treatment as even those who attended the outpatient clinics for weighing did not necessarily attend behaviour therapy groups or collect their drugs from the pharmacy. Continued attendance may only reflect commitment to treatment rather than compliance with prescribed behaviours. Nevertheless the existence of better attendance rates in behavioural than in other studies suggests that elements of behavioural therapy are contributing to enhance commitment at least at some level.

165

Contracts and financial reward

One method that appears to influence compliance in behavioural studies is the use of contracts, usually with a financial contingency. Contingency contracting involves an agreement between therapist and client on a reward-penalty system that is contingent on the client's weight changes. The client deposits some money or valuables with the therapist that are earned back or permanently lost. The problem here is that without learning habit change techniques as well subjects tend to regain weight when the contingencies are removed, so that this kind of system should only be used in conjunction with other strategies for inducing control.

Some 60 per cent of contracts are written, and most (74 per cent) are not negotiated but the conditions are determined by the therapist. These factors may have an important effect on outcome which, however, is as yet unknown (Kirschenbaum and Flanery, 1983).

An examination of several of the studies including a contract condition may, however, tell us something about the effect of financial contingencies on aspects of compliance.

Vincent, Schiavo and Nathan (1976) required their patients to deposit $5 'for materials', plus 0.5 per cent of net monthly combined income refundable contingent on attendance, punctuality, completion of weekly data forms, and habit change exercises. Patients in this group did no better than those in a self-management alone programme however, and both groups lost weight. Drop-out was 24 per cent for both groups.

Jeffery, Thompson and Wing (1978a) suggested that the failure of this and other studies to erase attrition was in their charging inadequate sums of money, and in putting the emphasis on attendance rather than on weight or habit change. They charged each subject in three contract conditions (weight, calorie and attendance) $200. In a ten-week programme, $20 were returned per week for a 21lb weight loss, for keeping within specified calorie limits according to self-report, or for attendance. Only 31 per cent of the original callers agreed to participate (having heard the conditions!) and only just over half of these turned up for the first session, but all subjects completed the requisite number of sessions compared to a control group formed from people who had declined the contract condition. The weight contract and calorie contract groups lost significantly more than the attendance contract group (about 20lb compared with 9lb and for the no-contract group, 12lb). Subjects in all conditions continued to lose weight on their own.

The problem with charging too large a sum of money is that this acts as a factor in ensuring that only the more highly motivated subjects will enter treatment in the first place. Subjects in Jeffery and colleagues' poorer outcome contract group did no better than subjects in the no-contract group (those who stayed). Presumably in this case the contract groups are simply differentiated from the other by being more highly selected from the start. Similarly, Harris and Bruner's (1971) contract group lost significantly more weight than self-control and control groups but only 5 out of 12 original recruits turned up for treatment, compared to 90 per cent of recruits in the self-control group. It may be that, contrary to Jeffery et al.'s suggestion, there is an optimum level of deposit for strengthening motivation without excluding all but the most highly committed subjects.

If there is an optimum level of financial contingency then the next question to be answered is that of what aspects of therapy the rewards should be contingent on. Heckerman and Prochaska (1976) extracted a $25 deposit from all of forty-three subjects in four treatment conditions. Subjects in the contingency contracting condition agreed to lose 2lb per week and to forfeit $2 of their deposit if they did not lose the weight and $2 for non-attendance. Subjects in a standard self-control and self-plus-internal control group were refunded $10 at the end of treatment. No subjects dropped out of the contract group, and there was 9 per cent attrition for the other groups. All experimental groups did better than controls (mean losses 10lb compared to a gain of 1.6lb by the control group). Losses were maintained at three-month follow-up and by 29 patients at one year. The finding that more frequent reward contingent on weight loss is more effective than a lump sum at the end has been confirmed in a more recent study with adolescents in which only those rewarded for loss on a daily basis lost a significant amount of weight compared with subjects rewarded only once a week (Coates et al., 1982).

Another fairly important factor is that of who does the

rewarding. Subjects who reward themselves out of their own deposits lose more weight than subjects rewarded similarly by the therapist (Mahoney, 1974; Jeffrey, 1974). Also reward for habit change is more effective than reward for weight loss (Mahoney, 1974; Kirschenbaum and Flanery, 1983). Overall, Jeffery and his colleagues (1984) have concluded that including contingency conditions in treatment results in an improvement over other treatments of 25 to 50 per cent.

Another aspect of contracts that may have implications for outcome is how public they are. Ureda (1980) included a weight control contract signed either by the participant alone or by a partner, friend or relative in a study which did not impose any formal system of reinforcement. The subjects whose contracts had been signed by someone other than the therapist did significantly better than the control group (although he did not state what the difference in weight loss was). Other studies that have involved a spouse or other significant person in the subject's life have increasingly supported the view that including family members in treatment has an important effect on compliance.

Including family members in treatment

Stuart and Davis (1972) noted that some husbands are 'not only not contributors to their wives' efforts to lose weight, but may actually exert a negative influence'. For those participants acknowledging receipt of help from another family member in reinforcing good eating habits, 83 per cent lost 20 per cent or more of body weight and maintained this for at least a year. Of participants who did not receive such help, only 31 per cent had similar success.

Becker and Green (1975) have reviewed the effects of families on their members' health actions *vis-à-vis* a range of medical problems, and cite four studies in which family members were seen to influence compliance with recommendations. For example, in a study by Heinzelmann and Bagley (1970) 80 per cent of men whose wives' attitudes towards a fitness exercise programme for coronary heart disease were positive, had good patterns of compliance. In relation to weight, Mahoney and Mahoney (1976) derived an index of social support based on family attendance and reports of co-operation and encouragement in a reduction programme which families were encouraged to attend. Scores on the index correlated significantly with weight loss.

There have been some recent attempts to explore the influence of family in a more controlled way. Wilson and Brownell (1978) compared the effects in an eight-week behavioural programme of having a family member present with not having a family member present. Family members were instructed to assist in monitoring, to reinforce improved eating habits, and not to criticise their partners. However there were no significant differences in results between the two conditions. One reason for this may be that no account was taken of the extent to which beliefs of family members about the importance of treatment were in concordance. Becker and Green (1975) report on a study by Becker and his colleagues (1975) of factors affecting participation in a Tay-Sachs screening programme. Where both husband and wife had low beliefs in susceptibility to or severity of being carriers of the gene, participation was lowest; inconsistent couple beliefs resulted in an intermediate rate of participation; and where joint beliefs were both in agreement and high, participation rate was highest.

Brownell and his colleagues (1978a) divided couples into treatment groups based on whether or not spouses wished to participate in the treatment as well. In a 'co-operative spouse couples' training group, spouses were given a manual and instructed to model and reward appropriate behaviours, and engage the subject in behaviours incompatible with eating. The couples were also instructed in mutual monitoring techniques. In another group subjects whose spouses had agreed to co-operate were treated alone; and subjects whose spouses had declined to co-operate were treated in a third group. Subjects in all groups lost weight during treatment, but at three and six months follow-up subjects in the couples training condition had lost significantly more weight than subjects in either of the other two conditions. Some support for these findings comes from other studies with similar conditions of spouse co-operation (Pearce *et al.*, 1981; Murphy *et al.*, 1982). There is some argument, however, as to the level of spouse co-operation actually required, and as to how far the active co-operation of a spouse contributes to long-term maintenance of weight loss. Thus for example the subjects with non-participating spouses in Pearce and his colleagues' study (1981) lost as much weight at post-treatment and at follow-up as did those whose spouses took an active part in treatment, and the authors suggested that instructing spouses not to interfere with their wives' weight loss attempts may have been as powerful as actually instructing them in behavioural self-control methods. Another study followed up married women whose husbands had to agree to involvement in treatment as a prerequisite to enrolment. Women who had attended treatment sessions alone lost significantly more weight at one year than those whose husbands had been passive observers at treatment sessions and did no better than women whose husbands had been actively involved in treatment (Black and Lantz, 1984). Possibly the key factor of importance in all these studies is that spouse co-operation, whether specific or not, is ensured, as opposed to active sabotage. In an interesting study which measured Expressed Emotion (Vaughn and Leff, 1976), Fischmann-Havstad and Marston concluded that wives whose husbands expressed most hostility and criticism of their wives in hour-long interviews on the subject of weight-reducing efforts were the most likely to relapse after successful weight reduction (Fischmann-Havstad and Marston, 1984).

Family involvement is also considered to be of key importance in relation to the treatment of obese children. In several studies Epstein and his colleagues have suggested that treating mothers in behavioural programmes together with their children results in good in-treatment losses and follow-up maintenance (Epstein *et al.*, 1980, 1981, 1984). Again what is important appears to be not so much the ability of the mothers to lose weight, but the kind of support they are able to give their children. In a study comparing different types of maternal involvement Brownell and his colleagues (1983) have shown that children whose mothers were treated in separate weight-reduction groups lost more weight and maintained their losses better at one year than did children whose mothers were treated in the same group or children who were treated alone; while in a more recent study children whose parents chose to learn 'helper' skills, including keeping records of specific behavioural changes and rewarding their child for completing homework assignments, maintained their weight as well as did children whose parents took part in weight reduction groups and were themselves rewarded for weight loss (Israel *et al.*, 1984).

Nutritional knowledge and expectations of weight loss

It could be said that involvement of families in weight control programmes has the effect of more widely disseminating knowledge about appropriate nutrition and more reasonable expectations of what the patient should lose. Ley and Spelman (1967) have proposed a cognitive hypothesis of patient satisfaction and compliance. They claim that non-compliance with therapeutic regimes stems from three inter-related facts. The first of these is that material presented to patients is often too difficult for them to comprehend. The second is that patients often lack elementary knowledge, and the third is that patients often have active misconceptions which mitigate against proper understanding. In addition, patients forget up to 50 per cent of information given to them by doctors as early as five minutes after a consultation. Increasing the reading ease of written communications, repetitions, and the use of concrete specific rather than general statements are all tactics that have been used with some success; and all are usually embodied in behavioural approaches to treatment. In relation to knowledge about diet and food values there does appear to be some evidence that the better people are acquainted with appropriate diet and nutrition, the more successful they are likely to be at dieting (Ley *et al.*, 1975; Brownell *et al.*, 1978; Dash and Brown, 1977). Of course this is only one factor in the complex mix of factors that relate to how likely an individual is to lose weight, but it is clearly worth including a strong educational element in programmes, as for example Ley (1976) found when subjects given an easy version of a leaflet designed to motivate them to keep to a diet lost nearly twice as much weight as a group given a more difficult version of the same leaflet.

Expectations about treatment itself are also important. In his summary of factors associated with compliance Haynes (1976) noted that many studies suggested an association between inappropriate health beliefs or expectations and compliance. In relation to the world of diet, inappropriate expectations must surely be fairly rife. The popular press abounds with diets

171

which claim spectacular weight losses within a few days and many people attending outpatient clinics admit to expectations of being able to lose far in excess of a kilogram per week. Ford and his colleagues (1977) found that subjects most in excess of their ideal weights held the least realistic concepts of expected rate of weight loss, and previous attendance at a clinic or slimming club had made no difference to this. Rodin and her colleagues (1977) noted that patients who felt that poor eating habits were an important cause of overweight lost twice as much as those who denied this; and patients who felt that hereditary or physical factors were of primary importance lost only half as much weight as those who did not. An assumption of behavioural treatment in particular is that patients' inappropriate expectations should be corrected if treatment is to be successful. This is an aspect of treatment that may require more empirical study in the future.

Related to the aspect of how to go about losing weight is that of information that the client may have about how important it is to him personally to weigh less. Becker and Maiman in their 'Health Belief Model' have suggested on the basis of evidence from other health fields that one of the elements contributing to a subject's willingness to take action is his perception of the probable severity of the disease (Becker and Maiman, 1975). In relation to obesity, however, those people whose main reason for losing weight is physical respond no better to treatment than do those whose main reason is psychological (Douglas *et al.*, 1981).

There have been one or two attempts to manipulate fear about the consequences of overweight in obese people in an attempt to increase compliance. For example Skilbeck and colleagues (1976) in an unpublished experiment reported by Ley (1976) found that whereas high, medium and low fear messages did not differ in their effects on weight loss, reported fear was associated with differences. Subjects who described themselves as moderately frightened by the experimental communication lost more weight than those subjects who described themselves as highly or hardly frightened.

Nevertheless this line of research appears not to have been pursued. Increasingly health professionals are realising that the strength of the desire to lose weight may have little association with losses achieved in treatment. This is highlighted by the increasingly prevalent problem of binge-eating, which may occur in grossly overweight people alongside a desperate wish to eat less and lose weight.

In the face of this dilemma, the keen desire of some people to lose weight alongside an apparent inability to adhere to advice aimed at helping them to do so, many writers have addressed themselves to the question of prediction of outcome on the basis of personal characteristics of sufferers.

Predicting individual response to treatment

Obesity is only one of many disorders of interest to medical and related professions where compliance with treatment is less than perfect. Nevertheless much time and effort has been addressed to the question of what kind of people are unable to follow the apparently simple prescription to eat less.

In relation to whether males or females do better, it seems that males lose more both at treatment and at follow-up (O'Neil *et al.*, 1980). However there is in fact less evidence in relation to men than there is in relation to women so this conclusion must be tentative (Weiss, 1977).

The evidence about age of subjects and age of onset in relation to dieting success is equivocal. In one study the average age of people who dropped out of treatment was 38, while the mean age of a 'persister' group was 51 years (Silverstone and Cooper, 1972). In a similar group of patients, however, there was no relationship between age and weight loss (Vincent *et al.*, 1976). In relation to age of onset of obesity too, some studies report that earlier onset is predictive of greater success in losing and maintaining weight loss than late onset (Johnson *et al.*, 1976; Jeffery, Wing and Stunkard, 1978). On the other hand more studies report greater success in people who became obese after adolescence (McReynolds and Lutz, 1974; Silverstone and Cooper, 1972; Craddock, 1977; Colvin and Olson, 1983). Also it seems that the more often diets have been tried in the past, the less well people do with current diets (Mitchell and Stuart, 1984). There may be a behavioural explanation for these findings. The longer a person has been overweight, the longer he or she has been eating more than needed to achieve a lower body weight; and hence the greater the habit strength and the more difficult it is to adopt a new eating and exercise pattern.

Other writers have looked at the relationship of weight loss with various measures of personality. Unfortunately the picture is complicated by the variety both in the measures used and of subject samples. A few studies have suggested a relationship between low Neuroticism and success with weight loss (Craddock, 1977; Silverstone and Cooper, 1972). Others have not found any relationship between Neuroticism and weight loss (Vincent *et al.*, 1976; Gilbert and Garrow, 1983). Many workers have attempted to differentiate between good and bad losers on the basis of scores on the MMPI (Minnesota Multiphasic Personality Inventory); but again results are equivocal. Several others have used Rotter's Locus of Control Scale (Rotter, 1966). The scale assesses the degree to which a person perceives control of events as coming from his environment or from within himself. It has therefore been considered relevant to the study of weight reduction which requires the person to make very definite self-controlled actions in order to achieve his goal. There are various problems with the use of such a test, however, that might partly explain why results have been so variable. One problem suggested by Lefcourt (1976) is that the concept may not be generalisable across persons. For example there is evidence to suggest that black people perceive causality differently from white people. Another problem is that the questions on the scale refer to political/social attitudes – for example, 'As far as world affairs are concerned, most of us are the victims of forces we can neither understand nor control,' versus, 'By taking an active part in political and social affairs the people can control world events.' The predictive power of the scale may thus be diluted when it comes to areas of personal control such as eating behaviour. Another problem is that the locus of control for failure and success may be relatively independent from each other, in that people are not necessarily totally internally or totally externally controlled. Despite these reservations, several studies have reported a significant relationship between Rotter's IE and success (Cohen and Alpert, 1978; Ley *et al.*, 1975; Balch and Ross, 1974).

An interesting finding in one study was that while IE did not correlate with weight loss in either of two treatment groups, weight loss in the control group which had no treatment at all was significantly correlated with Internal control (Manno and Marston, 1972). Similarly Jeffrey and Christensen (1975) found no significant differences in Internal control between losers and non-losers in a behavioural therapy group but internally controlled subjects in a 'will-power' control group lost significantly more weight than externally controlled subjects. Possibly Internal control is a relevant variable where treatment is limited, but becomes less important when superseded by the power of a behavioural programme.

Several other studies, on the other hand, have reported no relationship of weight loss with Internal External control either with groups of college students (Bellack, Schwartz and Rozensky, 1974; Tobias and MacDonald 1977) or with outpatient groups (Rodin et al., 1977; Vincent et al., 1976).

What does seem to come out of these studies, however, is the importance of perceived control, which may or may not be related to Locus of Control per se. For example, Leon (1975) found no correlation of IE with weight loss of slimming club members; but there was a significant relationship between answers to the question 'Do you feel you have good self-control?' and weight loss at six months follow-up (p <0.02). Similarly in a more recent study, Weight Watchers were asked how likely they thought they were to lose weight or to drop out of treatment and every week those who would later drop out reported significantly less confidence that they would reach goal weight than those who remained; and people who stayed in treatment reported more perceived success than did people who dropped out (Mitchell and Stuart, 1984).

Personality variables, then, are not particularly helpful in relation to prediction of response to the treatment of obesity. There are, however, some behavioural variables which are more relevant. For example, people who make life-style changes such as taking more exercise do better than those who do not (Harris et al., 1980; Gormally et al., 1980; Miller and Sims, 1981; Katahn et al., 1982, and Wing et al., 1984b). As noted previously people who are able to make long-term changes in the way they eat do well.

Another group of people who do well are those who describe themselves as being able to avoid eating for emotional reasons (Palgi et al., 1983; Marston and Criss, 1984). In our own outpatient group women who described themselves on a questionnaire as eating for emotional reasons lost more weight subsequently than those who denied this (Gilbert and Garrow, 1983). In one other study frequent binge-eating was a predictor of success (Gormally *et al.*, 1980). These findings are somewhat puzzling, but may indicate that people who are prepared to admit to a problem are more able to find solutions than those who deny having problems at all. In other studies, however, binge-eating has been described as a predictor of poor outcome in behavioural treatment (Wilson, 1976; Keefe *et al.*, 1984).

These considerations raise the question of how far self-control on its own is adequate to the treatment of obesity, particularly in relation to overeating. Given also that success in treatment is mediated by expectations or by belief in one's ability to succeed with dieting, the inclusion of cognitive therapy techniques in treatment is a logical development.

Cognitive therapy techniques in the behavioural treatment of obesity

There is much evidence that eating behaviour is partly mediated by cognitive factors. The amount of food eaten may be affected by how much the person believes he or she has eaten already (see page 123). Seeing food or thoughts about food can be cues to eat, particularly in a person who is already deprived. Eating may be stress-induced, and in some people restraint may be abandoned in response to depressed mood or anxiety or merely in response to having eaten too much already (see Chapters 7 and 8).

In an attempt to deal with these problems, some therapy programmes have included cognitive techniques for dealing with thoughts about food, guilt about having overeaten, and solving problems in relation to eating that cannot be dealt with by diet and stimulus control alone. For example the Mahoneys in their book *Permanent Weight Control*, have a chapter on 'Cognitive ecology: cleaning up what you say to yourself' (Mahoney and Mahoney, 1976). They suggest that dieters identify negative self-talk, for example excuses for overeating, setting unreasonably high goals, or thoughts about food. They suggest replacing 'negative monologues' with more appropriate ones. Thus, for example, the dieter who starts the day with a doughnut, instead of saying 'I've blown it for today, I might as well give up the diet' might tell herself that nobody is perfect, and one slip does not signify the end.

Other behavioural programmes now include cognitive strategies to a lesser or greater degree. In some cases this consists of giving guidance on specific positive thinking techniques to use and in others it consists of helping clients with more general problem-solving strategies. One approach which may have some applicability in this area is that of Beck *et al.* (1976). Garner and Bemis have described the possible use of Beck's cognitive therapy in relation to the treatment of anorexia nervosa (see Chapter 10), and have been able to identify thinking errors which are specific to anorexics. It should be feasible to conduct the same exercise in relation to obese people. This would be a particularly valid exercise if obese people are in fact depressed, but in any case is reasonable on the basis of the tendency for many obese people to feel negative about their image of their body and themselves or inadequate to the task of losing weight through dieting. Typical errors of thinking that will immediately be recognised by professionals used to working with dieters or overeaters are: 'discounting the positive' ('So what, I lost a pound this week. I should have lost six by now'); 'Catastrophising' ('If someone comments on my size I won't be able to stand it'); and 'all or nothing thinking' ('I've ruined my diet with that meal/cake. I might as well carry on eating'). Despite the apparent appeal of cognitive techniques as part of a programme of treatment in relation to overeating and obesity, few studies have tackled their merits relative to other techniques empirically. Two unpublished studies carried out as PhD projects in the late 1970s claimed good results with cognitive therapy in comparison to stimulus control with continuing losses at three-month follow-up in one study and only half the number of drop-outs in the other (Dono, 1976; Emery, 1979). In view of the inadequately substantiated connection between specific eating behaviours and overweight, this approach which addresses the beliefs, expectancies, self-image and motivation of people with chronic, perhaps intractable, health problems, merits further attention.

Another approach which addresses the cognitive aspects of dieting, and lapses in diet in particular, is that of 'relapse prevention'. The notion of relapse prevention is one discussed by Marlatt and Gordon. They investigated the characteristics óf situations in which alcoholics, smokers and drug addicts relapsed after treatment (Marlatt and Gordon, 1980). They ascertained that over half of all relapse situations occur either in response to frustration and anger, interpersonal or social, or in response to social pressure to resume the addictive behaviour. In the face of relapse the sufferer's state of mind is characterised by two elements. On the one hand he experiences dissonance between his perception of himself as an abstainer and the knowledge that he has failed to abstain; and on the other he attributes the cause of the transgression to internal weakness or personal failure. The additive effect of these two reactions increases the likelihood of repeating the restricted behaviour and going into 'full blown relapse'. Marlatt and Gordon suggest that clients should be specifically trained to guard against the possibility of relapse. Training should teach the client first to recognise high-risk situations likely to increase the risk of relapse: for example, to recognise situational cues, or cognitive strategies which might bring them closer to thinking about or engaging in the addictive behaviour; and to practise self-monitoring. Second, the client should be taught coping responses, such as being able to spend the evening in a bar without drinking, or in the case of food avoiding high-calorie snacks at a party, through *in vivo* training. Third, clients should be taught a general problem-solving approach which will give them skills for general relaxation, and for increasing feelings of control in making general life-style decisions. Fourth, the client should be taught about the negative long-term effects of returning to substance abuse in order to counter-act ideas about short-term enjoyment. Last, the client should be taught what to do if a slip does occur, so that one slip does not necessarily escalate into full-blown relapse.

The relapse prevention model is based on the assumption of addiction to the target substance. Its application to food must of necessity be very different from that to alcohol or drugs, which may have to be eschewed completely. Nevertheless, it may be reasonable to apply the model to those people in particular who have a preference for particular high-calorie foods, or for whom specific situations may trigger uncontrollable binge-eating. In one study, the addition of relapse prevention training to a behaviour therapy programme produced no better weight losses in the short term. However, with the addition of an intensive follow-up strategy, losses were maintained better over one year than they were in the group that received only behaviour therapy (Perri *et al.*, 1984a).

Clearly the addition of cognitive strategies to programmes for the treatment of obesity is a rational way to improve their individual outcome and credibility. How far they may potentiate the effects of stimulus control, however, is still in question. There is a difference also between cognitive strategies which are used to monitor thought cues to eating or self-reinforce for keeping to a diet, and those which may be used to deal with unrealistic expectations about weight-loss goals or negative thoughts about being fat. The former are extensions of stimulus control techniques. The latter, however, have more relevance to problem-solving and decision-making than to dieting *per se*. Strategies which implicitly question the dieter's reasons for wanting to lose weight, her view of herself as a fat person, and the question of permission to eat or to remain fat, may for some people lead inevitably towards a decision not to diet. In her book *Fat is a Feminist Issue*, subtitled *the anti-diet guide to permanent weight loss*, Orbach (1978) has advocated techniques which to some extent reflect those of cognitive therapy. The focus, however, is on the dieting itself rather than on transgressions of the diet. Instead of being advised to avoid 'forbidden' foods, dieters are encouraged to retrieve control over their eating by learning to sample them in limited amounts. They are taught awareness of the power of words like 'should'; and may be asked to consider giving up dieting in order to come to terms with the needs of their bodies without guilt and ultimately to eat less without the desire to starve or binge. The Wooleys have also expressed keen awareness of the suffering experienced by some grossly overweight people through repeated attempts to achieve weight loss through dieting, and have questioned the morality of encouraging all without exception to continue. They suggest that fat people be counselled in relation to their feelings about being overweight and their expectations of diet, and that they be given permission to consider the option of not dieting at all but of learning instead to live with the social and psychological burdens, the shame, that fatness brings with it (Wooley *et al*, 1979; Wooley and Wooley, 1984). In their programme at the University of Cincinnati, they prepare patients for a realistic appraisal of the

179

likely effect of dieting through teaching about obesity, and the effects of diet on metabolism, and through discussion of previous diet experiences. Each person plays a major part in selecting her own goals based on these discussions, goals which may include restricting their diet to a greater or lesser degree. The Wooleys have arrived at this form of individual treatment through the experience of watching the failure of many diet attempts and the pain thus caused.

What then are the psychological effects of dieting and of weight loss?

Psychological effects of dieting and weight loss

There can be little doubt that unsuccessful dieting has negative effects on mood for many people (see also page 90). Halmi and her colleagues (1980) have described the retrospective reports of patients who had undergone surgery for their obesity. The majority of these people claimed to have been preoccupied with food, irritable, anxious and depressed, whenever they had attempted to diet in the past. The diets were of course by the very nature of the subjects questioned, unsuccessful, and the same people reported less intense symptoms after surgery, many of them feeling elated and self-confident.

However, the effect of dieting on emotions is not uniform across all people. In our own outpatient study patients were asked to rate their moods on the Leeds scale for depression and anxiety (Snaith et al., 1976) at monthly intervals. It was remarkable that while for some people weight loss bore a linear relationship to anxiety, for some it bore a relationship to depression, for some it bore a relationship to both, while for others there was no relationship at all (unpublished data). Even where a relationship might be established, however, this does not give direction of causality; to find out which came first would require more detailed recording, possibly by daily rating of mood.

Several of the behavioural studies, however, have reported a generally positive association of improved mood with weight loss (Wing et al., 1984). Moreover there is no evidence to suggest that people drop out of behavioural programmes in response to increasing depression or that unfavourable reactions are a common problem.

Less is known about the psychological effects of other treatments, with the exception of operative procedures. Because of the mixed reception operative procedures have had, many researchers have spent time questioning patients after their operations. People whose operations were successful have claimed in interview to have greater self-esteem, and to be more socially active (Hall *et al.*, 1983; Halmi *et al.*, 1980). Other aspects do not appear to change so easily. Thus some writers have noted that the attitudes of many women to themselves or to their bodies remained negative for many years (Gentry *et al.*, 1984; Schiebel and Castelnuovo-Tedesco, 1977; Castelnuovo-Tedesco *et al.*, 1982).

Success in the treatment of obesity and overeating is mediated by a number of psychological and behavioural factors. Today's failed dieter may be tomorrow's patient. Whatever treatment is advocated will operate in company with a host of influences stemming from, among others, individual expectations, family pressures, and past experience. Any plan of treatment should take these factors into account, so that the would-be dieter can make an informed choice based on an appreciation of the difficulties inherent in engaging in treatment weighed against the likely rewards of being slimmer.

12   Treatment of bulimia

Binge eating is a poor predictor of response to the treatment of both obesity and anorexia nervosa. However, it is also experienced as a separate phenomenon. As more information has been gathered on the syndrome of bulimia or bulimia nervosa, it has become increasingly necessary to devise a treatment which is not merely an extension of that for either obesity or anorexia nervosa. On the whole, sufferers do not find appetite suppressants helpful (Fairburn, 1984); behavioural self-control has insufficient power; and inpatient restrictions akin to those prescribed for anorexics only postpone the problems until discharge.

Drug treatment

The first attempts at drug treatment of bulimics involved the use of anticonvulsants. Rau and Green (1975) claimed success in the treatment of fourteen out of eighteen patients with anticonvulsant medication, based on the finding of EEG abnormalities. Wermuth and his colleagues subsequently conducted a twelve-week double-blind crossover study comparing phenytoin with placebo (Wermuth *et al.*, 1977). Some of the patients reduced their binge-eating in response to the phenytoin, but the effect was not reversed in the placebo period, so that the authors were unable to conclude on the drug's mechanism of action. The results of these studies remain unconfirmed as other treatments with phenytoin have since been unsuccessful (Johnson *et al.*, 1983a).

An alternative treatment approach that has received some attention is an approach which utilises antidepressant drugs, based on the notion that bulimics are in fact suffering a form of depression (see Chapter 8).

Pope and his colleagues have reported on a controlled study

in which they randomly assigned twenty-two bulimic out-patients meeting DSM111 criteria, to either imipramine or placebo (Pope et al., 1983). The study was blind, and the patients were clearly unaware of which pills they were taking, as some of the placebo subjects experienced side-effects just as did some of those on active drug. By the sixth week of the trial, the nine patients in the drug condition had described a reduction in the number of binges experienced by 70 per cent, compared to a minimal reduction in the placebo group. The same patients also claimed a significant decrease in the intensity of binges, pre-occupation with food, and greater subjective 'global' improve-ment. They also had reduced scores on the Hamilton Rating Scale for depression (Hamilton, 1960) and these were corre-lated with the reduction in binge frequency. Seven of the subjects stopped binge-eating entirely and maintained their improvements for between one and eight months. On the strength of this study, the authors made antidepressant treat-ment the subject of a book optimistically entitled *New Hope for Binge-Eaters* (Pope and Hudson, 1984).

The results of other studies, while to some extent supportive of Pope and Hudson's work, have not been as conclusive. In a further study by the same authors, sixty five patients were treated with either tricyclic antidepressants or monoamine oxidase inhibitors (Pope *et al.*, 1983a). More than half of the patients reduced their numbers of binge episodes per week by over 50 per cent; but only one third stopped binge-eating altogether for a month or more and ten of the patients who did improve did so only after three or four successive trials of several drugs over several months.

More recently, Mitchell and Groat (1984) ran a controlled trial of amitriptyline with thirty-two bulimic outpatients. The measures they used were number of binge episodes per week, number of days on which binge-eating occurred, number of hours spent binge-eating, and numbers of vomiting episodes. On all these measures, the drug group did better than the placebo group, but the differences were not significant, as both groups in fact improved. The patients who were depressed at the start of treatment improved significantly less than did those who were not, but they also had higher initial symptom levels, and so the authors suggested that depressed people may have a poorer prognosis than do non-clinically depressed bulimics.

Other writers have advocated the use of the monoamine oxidase inhibitors in the treatment of bulimia. All six patients in one uncontrolled trial of phenelzine were said to respond 'dramatically' after three to fifteen years of illness, and subsequent to the failure of several other treatments, mainly 'psychotherapy' (Walsh *et al.*, 1982). In a further trial, the same group followed ten successful patients out of an original twelve, and noted that three relapsed after two to three months while five still needed to take the drug (Stewart *et al.*, 1984).

The same authors also conducted a ten-week double blind study which underlined the problems inherent in prescribing MAOIs for some bulimics who cannot keep to the dietary restrictions. Three subjects were dropped before the start of the study because of inability to keep to the diet; two were dropped during the study because of intolerable side-effects. Five out of the nine patients who did manage to stay on the active drug stopped binge-eating entirely, but three relapsed again after stopping the treatment (Walsh *et al.*, 1984).

Brotman and his colleagues (1984) have reviewed the treatment of twenty depressed bulimic patients considered to be on therapeutic doses of antidepressant medication at the Eating Disorders Unit of Massachussetts General Hospital. Thirteen of the subjects reduced their binge frequency by at least 50 per cent. Twenty-three per cent of the sample did not relapse but six months later were still on medication. Herzog (1984a) has noted that the drug doses used were not therapeutic and that the study may in fact have underestimated the power of antidepressant medication.

In conclusion, it seems that pharmacotherapy may hold some promise for the treatment of bulimia; but this implies an ability to take the drugs and maintain a therapeutic dose despite the problems of bingeing and purging, and that patients are able to adhere to prescribed diets. Even if drug treatment is effective in the short term, there remains the problem of what happens after one year or two post therapy, and of how long patients can be expected to continue on medication.

Herzog (1984a), while clearly convinced of the power of medication, has suggested on the basis of a review of all available drug treatments that 'pharmacotherapy should only be prescribed as part of a multimodal treatment approach that included medical follow-up and psychotherapy' (p.923).

Behaviour therapy

What then, has psychotherapy to offer the bulimic? As already noted in Chapter 11, it is difficult to assess the efficacy of psychotherapy in the treatment of overeating. The term 'psychotherapy' often embraces a variety of different verbal therapies, sometimes in combination. Because most has been written in relation to largely behaviourally oriented studies, these studies will be the main focus of the following section.

As with the therapies for obesity, behavioural therapy of binge-eating has taken various forms. Several of the treatments have been uncontrolled studies of therapy with one or two subjects. Earlier treatments used aversion techniques. For example Wijesinghe (1973) reported successfully treating two patients, with remission of symptoms for one year; and Kenny and Solyom (1971) used a covert sensitisation technique whereby electric shock was paired with a visual image of compulsive eating and vomiting. However, as noted in Chapter 11, the use of aversive treatment has not been pursued in relation to disorders of eating.

More recently, compulsive eating and vomiting have been treated by exposure and response prevention or delay, based on the idea that the vomiting, like the compulsive behaviour of obsessionals, is anxiety-reducing and therefore maintains the overeating. Thus Welch (1979) instructed his patient to confront intrusive thoughts about food with 'rational argument'. At each step in the forced vomiting response chain, the patient was asked to stop and delay the next action: for example to wait after finding a toilet before going inside; to wait after bending over the bowl before vomiting. With each successful week the time periods of delays were increased. Welch reported success with stopping the vomiting eight weeks into therapy and at follow-up of eleven months.

Rosen and Leitenberg (1982) used a more active response prevention technique, combined with exposure to target foods in five patients. Two out of the 5 patients had stopped vomiting at six months, 2 had improved but 1 was unchanged. Using a similar programme with fee-paying patients, Giles, Young and Young (1985) claimed significant reductions in binge-purge episodes for 20 out of 34 women with severe bulimia.

Linden (1980) added stimulus control and the development

of alternative incompatible responses to the use of response delay in the treatment of a bulimic of four years' standing. Binge-eating was decreased from six times per week pre-treatment to none by week nine, with maintenance of the improvement at six months.

The problem with most of these strategies is that they rely very much on the compliance of the sufferer. This of course is the major difficulty of the person who has been trapped in a cycle of binge-eating and purging for some considerable time. In my own experience, some bulimics find themselves unable to delay vomiting once they have binged, at least near the beginning of treatment, for fear of putting on weight. They adamantly see the binge-eating as the problem – if we could get rid of that they say, the vomiting would no longer be necessary. Others have difficulty in delaying the binge itself, and some can be persuaded only with difficulty to monitor bulimic episodes, saying that to write it down only makes them feel worse when all they want to do is to forget that they have a problem at all.

Loro and Orleans (1981) have suggested one possible way round this problem in a paper in which they advocate the use of 'programmed' binge-eating. They suggest that a binge is pre-scribed, but with the demand that the patient eat in a predeter-mined fashion – slowly, in private, and concentrating on the taste of the food. In this way the binge episode can be reframed as a structured learning experience. During the binge the patient is asked to keep records of the calories consumed and the thoughts, feelings and behaviours preceding, accompanying and following the structured binge. The binge is then discussed in a follow-up session with the therapist twelve to twenty-four hours afterwards. In effect the therapy is a form of paradoxical intention. Loro and Orleans claim that the therapy cannot fail, as if the client complies with the instruction to binge her perceptions and feelings of self-control around binge eating will undergo inevitable change. If, on the other hand, she returns to the therapy session without having followed the instruction to binge, this too can be interpreted as evidence of control. Through the subsequent use of cognitive restructuring tech-niques, the client can then be helped to view his or her binge-eating behaviour as a habit under the control of antecedent and consequent events.

Fairburn (1981) has reported in detail on the use of a more

orthodox cognitive-behavioural approach with eleven patients with bulimia nervosa of from two to thirteen years' standing. During the eight weeks of the first part of the therapy, he concentrates on the use of traditional behavioural methods. Patients first monitor their eating, then are encouraged to restrict their eating to conventional mealtimes, using stimulus control techniques. Each session prescribes clearly defined behavioural goals. In the second phase of treatment, the therapy concentrates on identifying the circumstances under which loss of control (by now less frequent) occurs. The patient is taught to cope with these situations through training in problem-solving and in challenging and replacing 'maladaptive' thoughts (see also Chapter 10, page 146). The patient is also encouraged to expose herself increasingly to banned foods once more, for example by going out for meals or to buffet parties. Using these techniques, Fairburn claimed a reduction in the frequency of bulimic episodes to less than once a month in 9 out of the 11 patients. The mean duration of the treatment was 7 months with a range of 3 to 12 months. At twelve-month follow-up of 6 patients 1 was still bulimic, 1 had stopped binge-eating and vomiting altogether, and 4 were doing it once every two or three months, when under stress.

Similar successes have been reported by Long and Cordle (1982) and Grinc (1982) with clients treated with combinations of behavioural self-control procedures and cognitive restructuring. Long and Cordle (1982) lay particular emphasis on the treatment of the bulimic patient at an individual level. Increasingly, however, the emphasis has been towards group treatment.

One area of group treatment that merits some attention is the development of self-help women's groups with a feminist bias. Boskind-Lodahl and White (1978) treated thirteen self-confessed binge-eaters in a group with a strongly feminist orientation, combining behavioural techniques with role play and guided fantasy. Twelve patients completed the group, and of these ten reported a decrease in bingeing and purging behaviour, with four stopping altogether. Other self-help groups have been set up along similar lines, and in England the ideas have been further developed by Orbach (1978, 1982) (see also page 179). Many women are helped by this approach, but the lack of formal evaluation has so far made it difficult to compare with other approaches or to make this kind of therapy more widely available in the field of health care.

Other more behavioural treatments which are being evaluated still remain largely in the range of uncontrolled studies, albeit with pre- and post-therapy measurement attempts. Lacey (1983) randomly assigned thirty bulimics to ten weeks of treatment or to assessment only. In the treatment groups patients received half an hour of individual therapy plus one and a half hours of group therapy per week. Patients contracted to attend all sessions and to eat the 'prescribed diet', and also to eat three meals a day. This was the so-called 'behavioural' aspect of the programme, which was followed by 'insight directed psychotherapy'. During the programme twenty-four patients stopped bingeing and vomiting by the tenth session and a further four patients stopped within a month of the end of treatment. Most of the patients maintained their gains for up to one year. Interestingly, the therapy was conducted by 'paramedical staff', with 'no specialist training in group techniques', and this raises the question of what factors in the therapy may have resulted in such a remarkable improvement. Lacey himself remarked that the patients of their own accord tended to form themselves into self-help groups after the end of treatment. In addition, the contract to maintain weight on a specified diet may have been particularly important. If it is the case that binge-eating is induced by malnutrition resulting from severe caloric restriction or from fluctuating levels of blood sugar or insulin, then maintaining a well-balanced diet may be vital. Dalvitt-McPhillips (1984) has claimed a 100 per cent success rate with advising bulimics on a diet of at least 1400 calories made up of fresh or frozen foods, free of additives, alcohol, refined sugar or white flour. Such excellent results with dietary treatment need to be replicated, but they may contribute to an understanding of the success of a study which incorporated a strong dietary element.

In another study focussing on group therapy, Connors et al. (1984) also claimed that group cohesiveness was a vital component of therapy. Again one of the predictors of good outcome was eating more regular meals. The content of the groups themselves included education about the socio-cultural, emotional and physical factors associated with the binge-purge cycle; setting short-term goals, and teaching assertiveness, relaxation, and other coping strategies. During an eight-week treatment period, the number of bulimic episodes was halved and at follow-up ten weeks later there was on average a 70 per cent reduction in bulimic episodes compared with pretreatment levels. Three patients were symptom-free, eight had reduced the frequency of bulimic episodes by more than 50 per cent, and six had reduced them by between 30 and 50 per cent. In addition, there were significant positive changes in areas of psychological functioning including self-esteem, perceived control over binge-purge behaviour, and on subscales of the Eating Disorders Inventory.

It emerges, then, that short-term group treatment has a beneficial effect on the symptoms of bulimia nervosa and may also have a part to play in modifying associated attitudes towards eating, weight and self-image. It remains to be seen which aspects of therapy are those which are most effective in producing change, and in enhancing maintenance and continued change after the end of treatment.

Yates and Sambrailo (1984) divided their twenty-four bulimics into two groups, receiving slightly different treatments. In the first group, sixty minutes of once-weekly cognitive behavioural therapy was followed by specific behavioural instruction. This involved training in the use of stimulus control procedures, response delay of overeating and use of activities incompatible with binge-eating. In the second group, only the cognitive behavioural part of the programme was used; this included teaching about the effects of bingeing and purging, assertion training, relaxation training and cognitive restructuring with a focus on the difficulties perceived in change and worry about the possibility of weight gain. Sixteen of the women completed therapy. Seven of these had significant reductions in the frequency of their bulimic episodes, but there was no significant difference in response to therapy between the two groups. Nevertheless the overall frequency of bulimic episodes decreased significantly over time, and all the subjects became significantly less depressed and anxious and higher in self-esteem than they had been before treatment. Because not all the women benefited from treatment the authors themselves have questioned the utility of using only six weeks of therapy, and it is clear from other studies that up to three or even seven months may be needed in order to achieve complete remission.

A similar conclusion was reached by Schneider and Agras (1985) as a result of treating thirteen women over sixteen weeks, also with a combination of stimulus control and cognitive behavioural techniques. This was a modified replication of Fairburn's (1981) programme in a group setting. The subjects of the study were women with a self-reported average of twenty-four self-induced vomiting episodes per week. After treatment, the number of vomiting episodes had decreased to an average of 2.2 times per week. The changes were accompanied by overall increases in the amount and frequency of food intake and the women described themselves as less depressed, and with lower scores on the Eating Attitudes Test. Six of the women maintained their improvements at six months, with five of these having ceased vomiting altogether. Five other women had, however, begun to increase the frequency of bulimic episodes since the end of treatment.

On the basis of these studies, it seems reasonable to conclude that cognitive behaviour therapy is an effective strategy for some patients with bulimia nervosa, often of long standing. It appears to work better the longer the period of treatment; and while there is some benefit in conducting therapy in a group format because of the peer co-operation engendered, individual sessions may have the advantage of defending better against the possibility of relapse.

It is less clear which other aspects of therapy in particular are the most effective. A comparison of successful group programmes reveals large apparent differences in content from one to the next: for example Lacey's (1983) programme, with its move from behavioural to 'psychodynamic' techniques, sounds very different from the strictly cognitive behavioural programme of Schneider and Agras (1985). In one controlled study, cognitive behavioural treatment was significantly more effective than a credible non-directive condition (Kirkley et al., 1985). Conversely in another study, individual behaviour therapy, cognitive behaviour therapy and an educational group therapy all produced equivalent improvements in the frequency of binging and purging (Freeman et al., 1985). It is feasible that there are more similarities in the content of programmes in terms of their degree of directive focus than appears, and it may be that if more writers were to describe in detail what they actually do in therapy, the common factors would emerge more clearly.

Nevertheless, cognitive strategies alone may not suit all bulimics. As stated earlier, not everyone finds it easy to identify dysfunctional thought preceding a binge. This was the finding also of Rossiter and Wilson (1985) in a single case crossover study of cognitive restructuring and exposure with vomiting prevention. The cognitive restructuring had a more rational appeal for subjects but was less effective than the more disliked exposure with vomiting prevention. These authors suggested that binge-eating may be one of those affective reactions (Rachman, 1981) that are unavailable for scrutiny; that the emotion comes before the thought and hence the only way to effect change is to attack symptoms directly rather than attempt to do so indirectly through cognitions. A further study by the same group lends support to these ideas. Seventeen bulimics were treated with either cognitive restructuring or a combination of cognitive restructuring plus exposure and vomit prevention. The combined treatment resulted in more significant reductions in binge-ing and vomiting post-treatment and in superior maintenance at one-year follow up (Wilson *et al.*, 1986).

The cognitive therapy approach makes sense in relation to theories of bulimia which take into account socio-cultural pressures and the concept of restraint, both of which may be available to cognitive mediation. If, on the other hand, binge-eating is largely stress induced, then possibly only a treatment which also directly attacks anxiety, such as response prevention, will be effective. Similar considerations may apply also in relation to the efficacy of drug therapy for some people.

However, as Rossiter and Wilson (1985) have pointed out, a major problem involved in treating bulimics is that they are often difficult to engage in treatment. Compliance with instructions for either behavioural or purely cognitive tasks alike may vary from one patient to the next. Possibly a combined drug and cognitive behavioural approach would be one way of overcoming this particular difficulty for some people. For the long term, however, attitudinal and behavioural change is essential. In relation to obesity, patients treated with behaviour therapy alone may be more resistant to relapse than those treated in combination with drug therapy. The answer may lie in the form of a cognitive behavioural intervention the shape of which may need to be tailored to the individual – an intervention the precise nature of which has yet to be determined.

13   Conclusions

Undereating and overeating are determined and maintained by a host of factors both psychological and environmental. Some of these are pressures which are peculiar to modern industrialised society. An increase in the variety, the palatability and availability of food may combine with 'hidden' ingredients to shape tastes and appetites on a wide scale. Our palates are tempted from all sides by the media to sample foods of increasing sophistication and needing decreasing degrees of preparation. It is now apparent that many of us eat in response to environmental cues such as the time of day or the mere presence of food. It is not surprising that at a time when we need to expend less energy, average weights in the Western world are on the increase.

At the same time we are in the paradoxical situation of being cautioned against excessive weight, and to be obese is to court shame, particularly for women. At a time when weight is on the increase the ideal image as advertised by the media is one of increasing slimness. There is evidence that many women are aware of this pressure. Many women of normal weight admit to feeling guilty about consuming quite normal amounts of food. Many also believe that they should be slimmer and the prevalence of both dieting and self-confessed overeating is on the increase.

It is difficult to draw together the disparate themes in relation to the causation of pathologies of eating as discussed in this book; but one factor that many obese, normal weight and underweight people have in common is the attempt to control weight by dieting. While most people maintain their weight at a fairly constant level over several years, for others food restriction or 'dieting' is initiated as a conscious attempt to reduce weight to what they consider is normal, a level which is largely culturally determined. As Polivy and Herman (1985) have pointed out in their discussion of dieting and bingeing, dieting is a purely 'cognitive' exercise. Its effects do not make it any easier for the dieter to maintain a lower weight for several reasons. First, metabolic rate is lowered so that the dieter needs to eat even less in order to maintain the lower weight or to continue to lose. Subsequent to dieting metabolic rate does not return quite to its previous level so that with successive diets the dieter may need to eat even less in order to lose weight (Garrow, 1978). Besides, contrary to what might be expected, some people in response to a transgression or believed transgression of the diet may eat more rather than less. This 'counter-regulation' effect which Herman and Polivy (1975) have observed in dieters of all weights, may be a factor which contributes to binge-eating in anorexics, normal weight and overweight bulimics alike. In addition, food restriction has been shown to result in overeating in otherwise normal people in response to starvation (Keys *et al.*, 1950). It is likely that there is a close connection between dieting and binge-eating. Binge-eating may for some people be an inevitable corollary of restriction, once set in motion. This may contribute to an explanation of why many diabetics, for example, under immense pressure to maintain a carefully controlled diet, may paradoxically experience dietary chaos. It raises the question of whether other people too, forced to observe certain dietary restrictions for health reasons, may experience similar as yet unreported problems.

No one theory alone provides a comprehensive explanation of the motivation of anorexics who are able to starve themselves to a dangerous level of malnutrition or of the differences between those people who are able to withstand the pangs of hunger and starve or diet themselves successfully and those whose control is punctuated with bouts of binge eating. One factor which all these people have in common is an unhappiness with their body image, and extremely poor self-esteem. It is feasible that in combination with the psychological and physiological stresses engendered by dieting, poor self-esteem in a setting of other environmental, competitive or family pressures may render the cognitive control or 'will power' needed for strict dieting impossible.

Much speculative theory has been put forward about the

psychopathology of both overeating and undereating. Still the evidence does not yet lend itself to an overall synthesis of causation.

Psychological techniques, and behavioural techniques in particular, have recently contributed to the treatment of eating disorders in several ways. First, they have contributed a series of techniques. Thus, for example, anorexics are persuaded more quickly to gain weight through contingency contracting, bulimics may be taught response prevention, and obese people are taught the techniques of stimulus control as a means of reducing intake. Knowledge about behavioural techniques is now widespread. Most dietitians include instructions to self-monitor in their advice about restricting intake. Techniques such as making food cues less salient by throwing away left-overs, keeping food in the freezer, are widely advocated by health professionals as well as by self-help and commercial group leaders. Increasingly behavioural techniques are also illustrated in the slimming 'press' along with instructions for new diets to be tried.

Nevertheless a problem which still exists is that there remains a myth that dieting is easy, the solution to being overweight is merely to eat less. Yet dieting is a difficult exercise, alien to most people and often the cause of problems with control not previously experienced.

As well as contributing to the available repertoire of techniques, behaviour therapy has made an important contribution in the area of compliance with treatment in that attrition is reduced not only in behavioural programmes but in relation to other techniques where the programme includes a behavioural element. In this respect, behavioural principles, and not merely techniques, are being utilised to obtain compliance with health care advice. An overall approach makes for more sense than an approach which merely extracts techniques and offers them as mechanical solutions. Thus, for example, behavioural principles have been used to devise programmes in relation to a variety of problems where the antecedents and consequences of a behaviour are taken into account in order to arrive at a possible solution. 'Children with life-threatening disorders such as rumination, or food aversions resulting in failure to thrive, have been treated successfully by means of behavioural interventions' (Lavigne et al., 1981; Handen et al., 1986). In relation to

Prader-Willi syndrome also, it has been possible through altering the rewards consequent on food stealing and overeating to engender self-control in two children and to maintain the improvement subsequently in their home environment with minimal supervision (Page *et al.*, 1983).

With the increasing use of cognitive therapy techniques in particular, it should become possible to extend the behavioural treatment of overeating and undereating to take into account more fully the many factors which contribute to trigger problems in self-control for the individual sufferer. If dieting is a cognitive, self-imposed exercise, restriction presents problems which are not only behavioural but also attitudinal and motivational. Such problems require a comprehensive approach to examine the antecedents and consequences, both behavioural and cognitive, of binge-eating and starving.

Group solutions are cost-effective, but in order to work most efficiently, behaviour therapy may need to be offered on an individual basis. For example, one elderly person may have different reasons for exhibiting a poor nutritional state from another elderly person. In the same way, different factors might contribute to a disorder of eating in a young anorexic or bulimic woman from those which produce disorder in another with the same symptoms. In order to arrive at an appropriate treatment it may be necessary to examine the meaning of the symptoms for each person, including setting factors, and antecedents and consequences of thoughts and actions alike.

Binge-eaters and excessive dieters are the casualties of a society which puts a premium on health, slimness, and the perfect body in a setting of abundant food. An alternative approach to treating the symptoms of the resulting pathology is in relation to better education and prevention. Negative attitudes to the obese, reduced activity in the absence of a decrease in food intake, and an obsession with health and fitness contribute to a dilemma which for some people vulnerable to disorders of weight may trigger dietary chaos or at worst chronic starvation.

Education in good nutrition and in particular in relation to establishing good eating and exercise habits in children without self-consciousness may help some families disposed to dietary problems to avoid obesity or the need to diet in the future. In addition there needs to be more discussion about the effects of dieting, its difficulties and its inherent dangers; so that those who do need to diet are better prepared for the inevitable difficulties and those who do not are less likely to try.

Bibliography

Abraham, S.F. and Beumont, P.J.V. (1982), How patients describe bulimia or binge-eating. *Psychological Medicine*, 12: 625–35.

Abramson, E.E. and Jones, D. (1981), Reducing junk food palatability and consumption by aversive conditioning. *Addictive Behaviors*, 6: 145–58.

Abramson, E.E. and Wunderlich, R.A. (1972), Anxiety, fear and eating: a test of the psychosomatic concept of obesity. *Journal of Abnormal Psychology*, 79: 319–21.

Abramson, R., Garg, M., Cioffari, A. and Rotman, P.A. (1980), An evaluation of behavioural techniques reinforced with an anorectic drug in a double-blind weight loss study. *Journal of Clinical Psychiatry*, 41 (7): 234–7.

Adams, N., Ferguson, J., Stunkard, A. and Agras, S. (1978), The eating behaviour of obese and non-obese women. *Behaviour Research and Therapy*, 16: 225–32.

Agras, W.S., Barlow, D., Chapin, H., Abel, G. and Leitenberg, H. (1974), Behavior modification of anorexia nervosa. *Archives of General Psychiatry*. 30: 279–86.

Agras, W.S., and Kraemer, H.C. (1984), The treatment of anorexia nervosa: do different treatments have different outcomes? *Eating and its Disorders*. ed. A.J. Stunkard and E. Stellar. New York, Raven Press, 193–297.

Allon, N. (1975), Fat is a dirty word: fat as a sociological and social problem. *Advances in Obesity Research: 1.* ed. A.N. Howard. London, Newman Publishing Ltd, 244–7.

American Psychiatric Association (1980), *Diagnostic and Statistical Manual of Mental Disorders*. 3rd edn, Washington D.C.

Anand, B.K. and Brobeck, J.R. (1951), Localisation of a 'feeding center' in the hypothalamus of the rat. *Proceedings of the Society of Experimental Biology in Medicine*. 77: 323–4.

Andersen, A.E. (1985), *Practical Comprehensive Treatment of Anorexia Nervosa and Bulimia*. London, Edward Arnold.

Ashby, W.A. and Wilson, G.T. (1977), Behaviour therapy for obesity: booster sessions and long-term maintenance of weight loss. *Behaviour Research and Therapy*. 15: 451–64.

Ashwell, M. and North, W. (1977), The prevalence of obesity in working populations in London. *Proceedings of the Nutrition Society*, 36: 109A.

Askevold, F. (1982), Social class and psychosomatic illness. *Psychotherapy and Psychosomatics.* 38: 256–9.

Baanders-van Halewijn, E.A., Choy, Y.W., Van Uitert, J. and de Waard, F. (1984), The Cordon study of weight reduction based on behavior modification. *International Journal of Obesity.* 8 (2): 161–70.

Baillie, P., Millar, F.K. and Pratt, A.W. (1965), Food and water intake and Walker tumor growth in rats with hypothalamic lesions. *American Journal of Physiology.* 209: 293–300.

Balagura, S. (1972), Neurophysiologic aspects: hypothalamic factors in the control of eating behavior. *Advances in Psychosomatic Medicine.* 25–48.

Balch, P. and Ross, A.W. (1974), A behaviourally oriented didactic group treatment of obesity: an exploration study. *Journal of Behaviour Therapy and Experimental Psychiatry*, 5: 239–43.

Baldry, J. (1981), Ethnocultural differences in preferred sweetness and firmness in mango and mango products. *Criteria of Food Acceptance: How Man Chooses What He Eats.* ed. J. Solms and R.L. Hall. Zürich, Forster Verlag AG, 138–42.

Baucom, D.H. and Aiken, P.A. (1981), Effect of depressed mood on eating among obese and nonobese dieting and nondieting persons. *Journal of Personality and Social Psychology.* 41 (3): 577–83.

Beauchamp, G.K. and Moran, M. (1982), Dietary experience and sweet taste preference in human infants. *Appetite: Journal for Intake Research.* 3 (2): 139–52.

Beck, A.T., Rush, A.J., Shaw, B.F. and Emery, G. (1976), *Cognitive Therapy of Depression.* New York, John Wiley & Sons.

Beck, A.T., Ward, C.H., Mendelson, M., Mock, J.E. and Erbaugh, J. (1961), An inventory for measuring depression. *Archives of General Psychiatry,* 4: 561–71.

Becker, M.H. and Green, L.W. (1975), A family approach to compliance with medical treatment: a selective review of the literature. *International Journal of Health Education.* 18: 2–11.

Becker, M.H., Kaback, M.M., Rosenstock, I.M. and Ruth, M.V. (1975), Some influences on public participation in a genetic screening programme. *Journal of Community Health.* 1(1): 3–14.

Becker, M.H. and Maiman, L.A. (1975), Sociobehavioural determinants of compliance with health and medical care recommendations. *Medical Care.* 13: 19–24.

Beidler, L.M. (1982), Biological basis of food selection. *The Psychobiology of Human Food Selection.* ed. L.M. Barker, Westport, Connecticut, Avi Publishing Co. 3–15.

Bellack, A.S., Schwartz, J. and Rozensky, R.H. (1974), The contribution of external control to self-control in a weight reduction program. *Journal of Behavior Therapy and Experimental Psychiatry.* 5: 245–9.

Bellisle, F. and Le Magnen, J. (1981), The structure of meals in humans:

eating and drinking patterns in lean and obese subjects. *Physiology and Behavior*. 27 (4): 649–58.

Beneke, W.M. and Paulsen, B.K. (1979), Long-term efficacy of a behavior modification weight loss program: a comparison of two follow-up maintenance strategies. *Behavior Therapy* 10(1): 8–13.

Ben-Tovim, D.I., Marilov, V. and Crisp, A.H. (1979), Personality and mental state (PSE) within anorexia nervosa. *Journal of Psychosomatic Research*. 23 (5): 321–5.

Bernstein, I.L. and Sigmundi, R.A. (1980), Tumor anorexia: a learned food aversion? *Science*. 209 (4454): 416–18.

Bernstein, I.L. and Webster, M.M. (1980), Learned taste aversions in humans. *Physiology and Behavior*. 25: 363–6.

Beumont, P.J.V., George, G.C.W. and Smart, D.E. (1976), 'Dieters' and 'vomiters and purgers' in anorexia nervosa. *Psychological Medicine*. 6: 617–22.

Bhanji, S. (1979), Anorexia nervosa: physicians' and psychiatrists' opinions and practice. *Journal of Psychosomatic Research*. 23 (1): 7–11.

Bhanji, S. and Thompson, J. (1974), Operant conditioning in the treatment of anorexia nervosa: a review and retrospective study of 11 cases. *British Journal of Psychiatry*. 124: 166–72.

Bigelow, G.E., Griffiths, R.R., Liebson, I. and Kalliszak, E. (1980), Double-blind evaluation of reinforcing anorectic actions of weight control medications. *Archives of General Psychiatry*. 37 (10): 1118–1123.

Birch, L.L. (1981), Generalisation of a modified food preference. *Child Development*. 52: 755–8.

Birch, L.L. and Marlin, D.W. (1982), 'I don't like it: I never tried it': effects of exposure on 2 year old children's food preferences. *Appetite: Journal for Intake Research*. 3: 353–60.

Birch, L.L., Marlin, D.W. and Potter, J. (1984), Eating as the 'means' activity in a contingency: effects on young children's food preference. *Child Development*. 55(2): 431–9.

Birch, L.L., Zimmerman, S.I. and Hind, H. (1980), The influence of social-affective context on the formation of children's food preferences. *Child Development*. 51 (3): 856–61.

Björvell, H. and Rössner, S. (1985), Long term treatment of severe obesity: four year follow up of results of combined behavioural modification programme. *British Medical Journal* (Clinical Research). August 10; 291 (6492): 379–82.

Black, D.R. and Lantz, C.E. (1984), Spouse involvement and a possible long-term follow-up trap in weight loss. *Behaviour Research and Therapy*. 22 (5): 557–62.

Black, D.R. and Scherba, D.A. (1983), Contracting to problem solve versus contracting to practice behavioral weight loss skills. *Behavior Therapy*. 14 (1): 100–9.

Blackman, S.L., Singer, R.D. and Mertz, T. (1983), The effects of social setting, perceived weight category and gender on eating behavior. *Journal of Psychology*. 144: 114–22.

Blinder, B.J., Freeman, D.M.A., and Stunkard, A.J. (1970), Behavior therapy of anorexia nervosa: effectiveness of activity as a reinforcer of weight gain. *American Journal of Psychiatry*. 126: 1093–8.

Blundell, J.E. (1980), Pharmacological adjustment of the mechanisms underlying feeding and obesity. *Obesity*. ed. A.J. Stunkard. Chicago, W.B. Saunders. 182–207.

Blundell, J.E. and Hill, A.J. (1985), Analysis of hunger: interrelationships with palatability, nutrient composition and eating. *Recent Advances in Obesity Research: IV.* ed. J. Hirsch and T.B.Van Itallie. London, Paris, John Libbey. 118–29.

Bo-Linn, G.W., Santa Ana, C.A., Morawski, S.G. and Fordtran, J.H. (1983), Purging and calorie absorption in bulimic patients and normal women. *Annals of Internal Medicine*. 99 (1): 14–17.

Bolocofsky, D.N., Spinler, D. and Coulthard-Morris, L. (1985), Effectiveness of hypnosis as an adjunct to behavioral weight management. *Journal of Clinical Psychology*. 41 (1): 35–41.

Booth, D.A. (1982), Starch content of ordinary foods associatively conditions human appetite and satiation, indexed by intake and eating pleasantness of starch-paired flavours. *Appetite: Journal for Intake Research*. 3: 163–84.

Boskind-Lodahl, M. and White, W.C. (1978), The definition and treatment of bulimarexia in college women – a pilot study. *Journal of the American College of Health Association*. 27 (2): 84–7.

Braitman, L.E., Adlin, E.V. and Stanton, J.L. Jr (1985), Obesity and caloric intake: the National Health and Nutrition Examination survey of 1971–1975 (HANES I). *Journal of Chronic Diseases* 38(9): 727–32.

Brala, P.M. and Hagen, R.L. (1983), Effects of sweetness perception and caloric value of a preload on short-term intake. *Physiology and Behavior*. 30: 1–9.

Branch, H. and Eurmann, L.J. (1980), Social attitude toward patients with anorexia nervosa. *American Journal of Psychiatry*. 137 (5): 631–2.

Brandon, S. (1970), An epidemiological study of eating disturbances. *Journal of Psychosomatic Medicine*. 14: 253–7.

Bray, G.A. (1981), The inheritance of corpulence. *The Body Weight Regulatory Systems: Normal and Disturbed Mechanisms*. ed. L.A. Cioffi, W.P.T. James and T.B. van Itallie. New York, Raven Press, 185–95.

Bray, G.A. (1984), Hypothalamic and genetic obesity: an appraisal of the autonomic hypothesis and the endocrine hypothesis. *International Journal of Obesity*. 8. Suppl. 1: 119–37.

Bray, G.A. and Gallagher, T.F. (1975), Manifestations of hypothalamic obesity in man: a comprehensive investigation of eight patients and a review of the literature. *Medicine* (Baltimore). 54 (4): 301–30.

Brewin, T.B. (1980), Can a tumour cause the same appetite perversion or taste changes as a pregnancy? *Lancet*. Oct. 25: 2 (8200): 907–8.

Brightwell, D.R., Foster, D. and Lee, S. (1980), Three-year follow up of subjects treated in a combined behavioral and anorectic weight control program. Paper given at International Congress on Obesity in Rome.

Brightwell, D.R. and Naylor, C.S. (1979), Effects of a combined behavioral and pharmacologic program on weight loss. *International Journal of Obesity*. 3: 141–8.

Brooke, C.G.D., Huntley, R.M.C. and Slack, J. (1975), Influence of heredity and environment in determination of skinfold thickness in children. *British Medical Journal*. 2: 719–21.

Brotman, A.W., Herzog, D.B. and Woods, Scott W. (1984), Antidepressant treatment of bulimia: the relationship between bingeing and depressive symptomatology. *Journal of Clinical Psychiatry*. 45: 7–9.

Brownell, K.D., Heckerman, C.L., Westlake, R.J. (1978), The behavioral control of obesity: a descriptive analysis of a large scale program. *Journal of Clinical Psychology*. 35(4): 864–9.

Brownell, K.D., Heckerman, C.L., Westlake, R.J., Hayes, S.C. and Monti, P.M. (1978a), The effect of couples training and partner co-operativeness in the behavioural treatment of obesity. *Behaviour Research and Therapy*. 16: 323–33.

Brownell, K.D., Kelman, J.H. and Stunkard, A.J. (1983), Treatment of obese children with and without their mothers: changes in weight and blood pressure. *Paediatrics*. 71: 515–23.

Brownell, K.D. and Stunkard, A.J. (1978), Behaviour therapy and behavior change: uncertainties in programmes for weight control. *Behaviour Research and Therapy*. 16 (4): 301.

Brownell, K.D., Stunkard, A.J. and McKeon, P.E. (1985), Weight-reduction at the work-site: a promise partially fulfilled. *American Journal of Psychiatry*. 142 (1): 47–52.

Bruch, H. (1962), Perceptual and conceptual disturbances in anorexia nervosa. *Psychosomatic Medicine*. 24: 187–94.

Bruch, H. (1974), *Eating Disorders: Anorexia, Obesity and the Person Within*. London and Boston, Routledge & Kegan Paul.

Bruch, H. (1974a), Perils of behavior modification in the treatment of anorexia nervosa. *Journal of the American Medical Association*. 230: 1419–22.

Bruch, H. (1977), Psychotherapy in eating disorders. *Canadian Psychiatric Association Journal*. 22 (3): 102–8.

Bruch, H. (1983), Psychotherapy in anorexia nervosa and developmental obesity. *Eating and Weight Disorders*, V. 8. ed. R.K. Goodstein. Springer, New York. 134–46.

Brummer, A. and Pudel, V.E. (1981), An attempt to demonstrate salivary increases in the hungry state. *Appetite: Journal for Intake Research*. 2: 376–9.

Buchwald, H. (1980), True informed consent in surgical treatment of morbid obesity. *Americal Journal of Clinical Nutrition*. 33: 482–94.

Bull, R.H., Engels, W.D., Engelsmann, F. and Bloom, L. (1983), Behavioural changes following gastric surgery for morbid obesity: a prospective, controlled study. *Journal of Psychosomatic Research*. 27 (6): 457–67.

Burns, T. and Crisp, A.H. (1984), Outcome of anorexia nervosa in males. *British Journal of Psychiatry*. 145: 319–25.

Button, E.J., Fransella, F. and Slade, P.D. (1977), A reappraisal of body perception disturbance in anorexia nervosa. *Psychological Medicine*. 7: 235–43.

Button, E.J. and Whitehouse, A. (1981), Subclinical anorexia nervosa. *Psychological Medicine*. 11 (3): 509–16.

Buvat, J. and Buvat-Herbaut, M. (1978), [Misperception of body concept and dysmorphophobias.] *Annales Medico-Psychologiques*. 136 (4): 563–80.

Cabanac, M. and Duclaux, R. (1970), Obesity: absence of satiety aversion to sucrose. *Science* 168: 496–7.

Cabanac, M., Duclaux, R. and Spector, N.H. (1971), Sensory feedback in regulation of body weight: is there a ponderostat? *Nature*, 229: 125–7.

Caldwell, M.L. and Taylor, R.L. (1983), A clinical note on food preference of individuals with Prader-Willi syndrome: the need for empirical research. *Journal of Mental Deficiency Research*. 27 (1): 45–9.

Canning, H. and Mayer, J. (1966), Obesity: its possible effect on college acceptance. *The New England Journal of Medicine*. 275: 1172–4.

Cannon, G. and Einzig, H. (1983), *Dieting makes you Fat*. London, Century Publishing.

Cantwell, D.P., Sturzenburger, S., Burroughs, J., Salkin, B. and Green, J.K. (1977), Anorexia nervosa – an affective disorder? *Archives of General Psychiatry*. 34: 1084–93.

Carlson, E., Kipps, M. and Thomson, J. (1984), Influences on the food habits of some ethnic minorities in the United Kingdom. *Human Nutrition: Applied Nutrition*. 38A: 85–98.

Carter, P.I. and Moss, R.A. (1984), Screening for anorexia and bulimia nervosa in a college population: problems and limitations. *Addictive Behaviors*. 9: 417–19.

Casper, R.C., Eckert, D.E., Halmi, K.A., Goldberg, S.C. and Davis, J.M. (1980), *Archives of General Psychiatry*. 37: 1030–5.

Casper, R.C., Halmi, K.A., Goldberg, S.C., Eckert, E.D. and Davis, J.M. (1979), Disturbances in body image estimation as related to other characteristics and outcome in anorexia nervosa. *British Journal of Psychiatry*. 134: 60–6.

Casper, R.C., Offer, D. and Ostrov, E. (1981), The self-image of adolescents with acute anorexia nervosa. *Journal of Pediatrics*. 98 (4): 656–61.

Castelnuovo-Tedesco, P., Weinberg, J., Buchanan, D.C. and Scott, H.W. Jr. (1982), Long-term outcome of jejuno-ileal bypass surgery for superobesity: a psychiatric assessment. *American Journal of Psychiatry*. 139 (10): 1248–52.

Celesia, G.G., Archer, C.R. and Chung, H.D. (1981), Hyperphagia and obesity. Relations to medical hypothalamic lesions. *Journal of the American Medical Association*. 246 (2): 151–3.

Charcot, J.M. (1889), *Diseases of the Nervous System*. London: The New Sydenham Society.

Chatoor, I., Dickson, L. and Einhorn, A. (1984), Rumination: etiology and treatment. *Pediatric Annals*. 13 (12): 924–9.

Chetwynd, S.J., Stewart, R.A. and Powell, G.E. (1975), Social attitudes towards the obese physique. *Recent Advances in Obesity Research I.* ed. A. Howard, London, Newman Publishing, 223–6.

Chiodo, J. and Latimer, P.R. (1983), Vomiting as a learned weight-control technique in bulimia. *Journal of Behavior Therapy and Experimental Psychiatry*. 13 (2): 131–5.

Cinciprini, P.M., Kornblith, S.J., Turner, S.M. and Hersen, M. (1983), A behavioral programme for the management of anorexia and bulimia. *Journal of Nervous and Mental Diseases*. 171 (3): 186–9.

Coates, T.J., Jeffrey, R.W. and Wing, R.R. (1978), The relationship between persons' relative body weights and the quality and quantity of food stored in their homes. *Addictive Behaviors*. 3 (304): 179–84.

Coates, T.J., Jeffrey, R.W., Slinkard, L.A., Killen, J.D. and Danaher, B.G. (1982), Frequency of contact and monetary reward in weight loss, lipid change, and blood pressure reduction with adolescents. *Behavior Therapy*. 13 (2): 175–85.

Cohen, N.L., and Alpert, M. (1978), Locus of control as a predictor of outcome in treatment of obesity. *Psychological Reports* 42(3): 805–6.

Collipp, P.J. (1984), Anorexia nervosa and binge vomiting. *Pediatric Annals*. 13 (7): 538–412.

Colvin, R.H., and Olson, S.B. (1983), A descriptive analysis of men and women who have lost significant weight and are highly successful at maintaining the loss. *Addictive Behaviors*. 8 (3): 287–95.

Connors, M.E., Johnson, C.L. and Stuckey, M.K. (1984), Treatment of bulimia with brief psychoeducational group therapy. *American Journal of Psychiatry*. 141 (12): 1512–16.

Cooper, P.J. and Fairburn, C.G. (1983), Binge-eating and self-induced vomiting in the community. A preliminary study. *British Journal of Psychiatry*. 142: 139–44.

Cooper, P.J. and Fairburn, C.G. (1984), Cognitive behaviour therapy for anorexia nervosa: some preliminary findings. *Journal of Psychosomatic Research*. 28 (6): 493–9.

Cooper, P.J., Waterman, G. and Fairburn, C.G. (1984), Women with eating problems: a community survey. *British Journal of Clinical Psychology*. 23: 45–52.

Coplin, S.S., Hine, J. and Gormican, A. (1976), Out-patient dietary management in the Prader-Willi syndrome. *Journal of the American Dietetic Association*. 68: 331–4.

Craddock, D. (1977). The free diet: 150 cases personally followed up after 10 to 18 years. *International Journal of Obesity*. 1: 127–34.

Craddock, D. (1978), *Obesity and Its Management*. 3rd edn. Edinburgh and London, Churchill Livingstone.

Craighead, L.W. (1984), Sequencing of behavior therapy and pharmacotherapy for obesity. *Journal of Consulting and Clinical Psychology*. 52(2): 190–9.

Crisp, A.H. (1966), A treatment regimen for anorexia nervosa. *British Journal of Psychiatry*. 112: 505–12.

Crisp, A.H. (1977), Diagnosis and outcome of anorexia nervosa. The St George's view. *Proceedings of the Royal Society of Medicine*. 70 (7): 464–70.

Crisp, A.H. (1981), Abnormal normal weight control syndrome. *International Journal of Psychiatry in Medicine*. 11 (3): 203–33.

Crisp, A.H., Fenton, G.W. and Srotton, L. (1968), A controlled study of the EEG in anorexia nervosa. *British Journal of Psychiatry*. 114: 1149–69.

Crisp, A.H., Harding, B. and McGuiness, B. (1974), Anorexia nervosa, psychoneurotic characteristics of parents; relationship to prognosis: a qualitative study. *Journal of Psychosomatic Research*. 18: 167–73.

Crisp, A.H., Hsu, L.K.G., Harding, B. and Hartshorn, J. (1980), Clinical features of anorexia nervosa. A study of a consecutive series of 102 female patients. *Journal of Psychosomatic Research*. 24: 179–91.

Crisp, A.H., Palmer, R.L. and Kalucy, R.S. (1976), How common is anorexia nervosa? A prevalence study. *British Journal of Psychiatry*. 128: 549–54.

Crisp, A.H., Queenan, M., Sittampaln, Y. and Harris, G. (1980a), 'Jolly Fat' revised. *Journal of Psychosomatic Research*. 24: 233–41.

Critchley, M. and Hoffman, H. (1942), The syndrome of periodic somnolence and morbid hunger (Kleine-Levin syndrome). *British Medical Journal*. 1 (4230): 137–9.

Dahlkoetter, J., Callahan, E.J. and Linton, J. (1979), Obesity and the unbalanced energy equation: Exercise versus eating habit change. *Journal of Consulting and Clinical Psychology*. 47 (5): 898–905.

Dahms, W.T., Molitch, M.E., Bray, G.A. and Greenaway, F.L. (1978), Treatment of obesity: cost-benefit assessment of behavioral therapy, placebo, and two anorectic drugs. *American Journal of Clinical Nutrition*. 31: 774–78.

Dally, P. (1969), *Anorexia Nervosa*. New York, Grune and Stratton.

Dally, P. and Gomez, J. (1979), *Anorexia Nervosa*. London, Heinemann.

Dally, P. and Sargent, W. (1966), Treatment and outcome of anorexia nervosa. *British Medical Journal*. 2:793.

Dalvitt-McPhillips, S. (1984), A dietary approach to bulimia treatment. *Physiology and Behavior*. 33: 769–75.

Dash, J.D. and Brown, R.A. (1977), The development of a rating scale for the prediction of success in weight reduction. *Journal of Clinical Psychology*. 33 (3): 748–52.

Dawes, M.G. (1984), Obesity in a Somerset town: prevalence and relationship to morbidity. *Journal of the Royal College of General Practitioners*. 34 (263): 328–80.

De Wys, W.D. (1978), Changes in taste sensation and feeding behaviour in cancer patients: a review. *Journal of Human Nutrition*. 32: 447–53.

Dodd, D.K., Birky, H.J. and Stalling, R.B. (1976), Eating behaviour of obese and nonobese females in a natural setting. *Addictive Behaviors*. 2: 321–5.

Dono, J.F. (1976), Effects of cognitive therapy and behavioral practice on weight reduction and locus of control. *Dissertation Abstracts International*. 37 (iB) 457.

Douglas, J.G., Ford, M.J. and Munro, J.F. (1981), Patient motivation and predicting outcome in a hospital obesity clinic. *International Journal of Obesity*. 5: 33–8.

Drenowski, A., Brunzell, J.D., Sande, K., Iverius, P.H. and Greenwood, M.R.C. (1983), Cream or sugar: obese subjects' preferences for sweetened high fat foods. Paper given at International Congress on Obesity in New York.

Drenowski, A. and Greenwood, M.R.C. (1983), Cream and sugar: human preferences for high-fat foods. *Physiology and Behavior*. 30: 629–33.

Duckro, P.N., Leavitt, J.N. Jr, Beal, D.G. and Chang, A.F. (1983), Psychological status among female candidates for surgical treatment of obesity. *International Journal of Obesity*. 7 (5): 477–85.

Dunn, J. (1980), Feeding and sleeping. *Scientific Foundations of Developmental Psychiatry*. ed. M. Rutter. London, William Heinemann. 119–28.

Durrant, M. (1981), Salivation: a useful research tool? *Appetite: Journal for Intake Research*. 2: 362–5.

Durrant, M. and Royston, P. (1979), Short-term effects of energy density on salivation, hunger and appetite in obese subjects. *International Journal of Obesity*. 3: 335–47.

Durrant, M.L., Royston, J.P., Block, R.T. and Garrow, J.S. (1982), The effect of covert changes in energy density of preloads on subsequent ad libitum energy intake in lean and obese human subjects. *Human Nutrition: Clinical Nutrition*. 36C: 297–306.

Eckert, E.D. (1983), Behavior modification in anorexia nervosa: a comparison of two reinforcement schedules. *Anorexia Nervosa: Recent Developments in Research*. ed. P.L. Darby, P.E. Garfinkel, D.M. Garner and D.V. Coscina. Alan R. Liss. New York, 377–85.

Eckert, E.D., Goldberg, S.C., Halmi, K.A. Casper, R.C. and Davis, J.M. (1982), Depression in anorexia nervosa. *Psychological Medicine* 12 (1): 115–22.

Edelman, B. (1981), Binge-eating in normal weight and overweight individuals. *Psychological Reports*. 49 (3): 739–46.

Emery, G.D. (1979), Cognitive versus behavioral methods in the treatment of overweight college students. *Dissertation Abstracts International*. 38 (11–B): 5563–4.

Epstein, L.H., Wing, R.R., Koeske, R., Andrasik, F. and Ossip, D.J. (1981), Child and parent weight loss in family-based behavior modification programs. *Journal of Consulting and Clinical Psychology*. 49: 674–85.

Epstein, L.H., Wing, R.R., Koeske, R. and Valoski, A. (1984), Effects of diet plus exercise on weight changes in parents and children. *Journal of Consulting and Clinical Psychology*. 52 (3): 429–37.

Epstein, L.H., Wing, R.R., Steranchak, L., Dickson, B. and Michelson, J. (1980), Comparison of family-based behavior modification and nutrition education for childhood obesity. *Journal of Pediatric Psychology*. 5 (1): 25–36.

Exton-Smith, A.N. (1980), Eating Habits of the Elderly. *Nutrition and Lifestyles*. ed, M.R. Turner. London. Applied Science Publishers Ltd. 179–94.

Fairburn, C. (1981), A cognitive behavioural approach to the treatment of bulimia. *Psychological Medicine*. 11: 707–11.

Fairburn, C.G. (1984), Bulimia: its epidemiology and management. *Eating and its Disorders*. ed. A.J. Stunkard and E. Stellar. New York, Raven Press, 235–58.

Fairburn, C.G. and Cooper, P.J. (1982), Self-induced vomiting and bulimia nervosa: an undetected problem. *British Medical Journal*. 284; 17 April. 1153–5.

Fairburn, C.G. and Cooper, P.J. (1984), The clinical features of bulimia nervosa. *British Journal of Psychiatry* 144: 238–46.

Falk, J.R. and Halmi, K.A. (1982), Amenorrhea in anorexia nervosa: examination of the critical body weight hypothesis. *Biological Psychiatry*. 17 (7): 799–806.

Feighner, J.P., Robins, E., Guze, S.B., Woodruff, R.A., Winokur, G. and Munoz, R. (1972), Diagnostic criteria for use in psychiatric research. *Archives of General Psychiatry*. 26: 57–63.

Ferster, C.B., Nurnberger, J.I. and Levitt, E.B. (1962), The control of eating. *Journal of Mathetics*. 1: 87–109.

Fischmann-Havstad, L. and Marston, A.R. (1984), Weight-loss maintenance as an aspect of family emotion and process. *British Journal of Clinical Psychology*. 23: 265–71.

Fitzgibbon, T. (1981), *The Pleasures of the Table*. Oxford, Oxford University Press.

Ford, M.J., Scorgie, R.E. and Munro, J.F. (1977), Anticipated rate of weight loss during dieting. *International Journal of Obesity*, 1: 239–43.

Foreyt, J.P. and Hagen, R.L. (1973), Covert sensitization: conditioning or suggestion? *Journal of Abnormal Psychology*. 82: 17–23.

Foreyt, J.P. and Kennedy, W.A. (1971), Treatment of overweight by aversion therapy. *Behaviour Research and Therapy*. 9 (1): 29–34.

Foreyt, J.P. and Kondo, A.T. (1984), Advances in behavioral treatment of obesity. *Progress in Behavior Modification*. 16: 231–61.

Freeman, C., Sinclair, F., Turnbull, J., Annandale, A. (1985), Psychotherapy for bulimia: a controlled study. *Journal of Psychiatric Research*. 19 (2–3): 373–8.

Freimer, N., Echenberg, D. and Kretchner, N. (1983), Cultural variation – nutritional and clinical implications. *Western Journal of Medicine*. 139 (6): 928–33.

Fries, H. (1974), Secondary amenorrhoea, self-induced weight reduction in anorexia nervosa. *Acta Psychiatrica Scandinavica*, Supplement 248.

Frijters, J.E. and Rasmüssen-Conrad, E.L. (1982), Sensory discrimination, intensity perception, and affective judgement of sucrose sweetness in the overweight. *Journal of General Psychology*. 107 (2): 233–47.

Frost, R.O., Goolkasian, G.A., Ely, R.J. and Blanchard (1982), Depression, restraint and eating behaviour. *Behaviour Research and Therapy*. 20: 113–21.

Garb, J.L., Garb, J.R. and Stunkard, A.J. (1975), Social factors and obesity in Navajo Indian children. *Recent Advances in Obesity Research,* vol. 1. ed. A.N. Howard. London, Newman. 37–9.

Garfinkel, P.E. and Garner, D.M. (1982), *Anorexia Nervosa: A Multidimensional Perspective*. New York, Montreal, Brunner/Mazel.

Garfinkel, P.E. and Garner, D.M. (1983), The multidetermined nature of anorexia nervosa. *Anorexia Nervosa: Recent Developments in Research*. ed. P.L. Darby, P.E. Garfinkel, D.M. Garner, D.V. Coscina. New York, Alan R. Liss. 3–14.

Garfinkel, P.E., Garner, D.M., Rose, J., Darby, P.L., Brandes, J.J., O'Hanlon, J. and Walsh, N. (1983), A comparison of characteristics in the families of patients with anorexia nervosa and normal controls. *Psychological Medicine*. 13: 811–28.

Garfinkel, P.E., Kline, S.A. and Stancer, H.C. (1973), Treatment of anorexia nervosa using operant conditioning techniques. *Journal of Nervous and Mental Disease*. 157: 428–33.

Garg, S.K. and Singh, S. (1983), Physiological basis of feeding behavior. *Personality Study and Group Behavior*. 3 (2): 1–20.

Garn, S.M. (1980), Human growth. *Annual Review of Anthropology*. 9: 275–92.

Garn, S.M., Bailey, S.M., Cole, P.E. and Higgins, I.T.T. (1977), Level of education, level of income and level of fatness in adults. *American Journal of Clinical Nutrition*. 30: 721–5.

Garn, S.M., Bailey, S.M. Solomon, M.A. and Hopkins, P.J. (1981), Effect of remaining family members on fatness prediction. *American Journal of Clinical Nutrition*. 34: 148–53.

Garner, D.M. and Bemis, K. (1982), A cognitive-behavioral approach to anorexia nervosa. *Cognitive Therapy and Research*. 6: 1–27.

Garner, D.M. and Garfinkel, P.E. (1979), The Eating Attitudes Test. *Psychological Medicine*. 9 (2): 273–80.

Garner, D.M. and Garfinkel, P.E. (1980), Socio-cultural factors in the development of anorexia nervosa. *Psychological Medicine*. 19 (4): 647–56.

Garner, D.M., Garfinkel, P.E. and Bemis, K.M. (1982), A multidimensional psychotherapy for anorexia nervosa. *International Journal of the Eating Disorders*. 1 (2): 3–46.

Garner, D.M., Garfinkel, P.E. and Olmsted, M.P. (1983), An overview of sociocultural factors in the development of anorexia nervosa. *Anorexia Nervosa: Recent Developments in Research*. ed. P.L. Darby, P.E. Garfinkel, D.M. Garner, D.V. Coscina. New York, Alan R. Liss, 65–82.

Garner, D.M., Garfinkel, P.E., Schwartz, D. and Thompson, M. (1980), Cultural expectations of thinness in women. *Psychological Reports*. 47 (2): 483–91.

Garner, D.M., Olmstead, M.P. and Garfinkel, P.E. (1985), Similarities among bulimic groups selected by different weights and weight histories. *Journal of Psychiatric Research* 19 (2–3): 129–34.

Garner, D.M., Olmstead, M.P., and Polivy, J. (1983), The eating disorder inventory: a measure of cognitive-behavioral dimensions in anorexia nervosa and bulimia. *Anorexia Nervosa: Recent Developments in Research*. ed. P.L. Darby, P.E. Garfinkel, D.M. Garner, D.V. Coscina. New York, Alan R. Liss. 173–84.

Garrow, J.S. (1978), *Energy Balance and Obesity in Man*. Amsterdam, Elsevier.

Garrow, J. (1978a), The regulation of energy expenditure. *Recent Advances in Obesity Research II*. Ed. G.A. Bray. London, Newman. 200–10.

Garrow, J.S. (1979), Weight penalties. *British Medical Journal*. 2: 1171–2.

Garrow, J.S. (1981), *Treat Obesity Seriously: A Clinical Manual*. Edinburgh, Churchill Livingstone.

Garrow, J.S. and Gardiner, G.T. (1981), Maintenance of weight loss in obese patients after jaw-wiring. *British Medical Journal*. 282: 858.

Gaul, D.J., Craighead, E. and Mahoney, M.J. (1975), Relationship between eating rates and obesity. *Journal of Consulting and Clinical Psychology*. 43 (2): 123–5.

Geiselman, P.J. and Novin, D. (1982), The role of carbohydrates in appetite, hunger and obesity. *Appetite: Journal for Intake Research*. 3 (3): 203–23.

Gentry, K., Halverson, J.D. and Heisler, S. (1984), Psychologic assessment of morbidly obese patients undergoing gastric bypass: a comparison of preoperative and postoperative adjustment. *Surgery* 95 (2): 215–20.

Gershon, E.S., Hamovit, J.R., Schreiber, J.L., Dibble, E.D., Kaye, W., Nurnberger, J.I., Andersen, A. and Ebert, M. (1983), Anorexia nervosa and major affective disorders associated in families: a preliminary report. In *Childhood Psychopathology and Development*. eds Guze, S.B., Earls, F.J. and Barrett, J.E., New York, Raven Press, 279–84.

Gershon, E.S., Schreiber, J.L., Hamovit, J.R., Dibble, E.D., Kaye, W.,

Nurnberger, J.I. Jr, Andersen, A.E. and Ebert, M. (1984), Clinical findings in patients with anorexia nervosa and affective illness in their relatives. *American Journal of Psychiatry*. 14 (11): 1419–22.

Gilbert, S. and Garrow, J.S. (1983), A prospective controlled trial of outpatient treatment for obesity. *Human Nutrition: Clinical Nutrition*. 37C: 21–9.

Giles, T.R., Young, R.R. and Young, D.E. (1985), Behavioral treatment of severe bulimia. *Behavior Therapy* 16: 393–405.

Glucksman, M.L. (1972), Psychiatric observations on obesity. *Advances in Psychosomatic Medicine*. 7: 194–216.

Glucksman, M.L. and Hirsch, J. (1968), The response of obese patients to weight reduction: a clinical evaluation of behaviour. *Psychosomatic Medicine*. 30: 1–11.

Gold, M.S., Pottash, A.L.C., Sweeney, D.R., Martin, D.M. and Davies, R.K. (1980), Further evidence of hypothalamic-pituitary dysfunction in anorexia nervosa. *American Journal of Psychiatry*. 137 (1): 101–2.

Goldberg, S.G., Halmi, K.A., Casper, R.C. and Davis, J.M. (1979), Cyproheptadine in anorexia nervosa. *British Journal of Psychiatry*. 134: 67–70.

Goldfarb, L.A. and Plante, T.G. (1984), Fear of fat in runners: an examination of the connection between anorexia nervosa and distance running. *Psychological Reports*. 55 (1): 296.

Goldfried, M.R. and Goldfried, A.O. (1975), Cognitive change methods. *Helping People Change*. ed. F.H. Kanfer and A.P. Goldstein. New York, Pergamon Press. 89–116.

Goodstein, R.K. (1983), *Eating and Weight Disorders*, New York, Springer.

Gormally, J. and Rardin, D. (1981), Weight loss and maintenance and changes in diet and exercise for behavioral counselling and nutrition education, *Journal of Counseling Psychology*. 28 (4): 295–304.

Gormally, J., Rardin, D. and Black, S. (1980), Correlates of successful response to a behavioral weight control clinic. *Journal of Counseling Psychology*. 27 (2): 179–91.

Gotestam, K.G. (1979), A three-year follow-up of a behavioral treatment of obesity. *Addictive Behaviors*. 4: 179–83.

Grace, P.S., Jacobson, R.S. and Fullager, C.J. (1985), A pilot comparison of purging and non-purging bulimics. *Journal of Clinical Psychology*. 41 (2): 173–80.

Graham, L.E. Taylor, C.B., Hovell, M.F. and Sitgel, W. (1983), Five-year follow-up to a behavioral weight loss program. *Journal of Consulting and Clinical Psychology*. 51 (2): 322–3.

Grinc, G.A. (1982), A cognitive-behavioral model for the treatment of chronic vomiting. *Journal of Behavioral Medicine*. 5: 135–41.

Grinker, J. (1978), Obesity and sweet taste. *American Journal of Clinical Nutrition*. 31 (6): 1078–87.

Gross, H.A., Ebert, M.H., Fader, V.B., Goldberg, S., Nee, L. and Kaye, W.

(1981), A double-blind controlled trial of Lithium carbonate in primary anorexia nervosa. *Journal of Clinical Psychopharmacology*. 1: 376–81.

Grossman, S.P. (1976), Neuroanatomy of food and water intake. *Hunger: Basic Mechanisms and Clinical Implications*. ed. D. Novin, W. Wyrwicka, and G. Bray. New York, Raven Press. 51–9.

Grossman, S.P. (1984), Contemporary problems concerning our understanding of brain mechanisms that regulate food intake and body weight. *Eating and its Disorders*. eds. A.J. Stunkard and E. Stellar. New York, Raven press. 5–14.

Grunewald, K.K. (1985), Weight control in young college women: who are the dieters? *Journal of the American Dietetic Association* 85 (11): 1445–50.

Gull, Sir W.W. (1874), Anorexia nervosa (apepsia hysterica, anorexia hysterica). *Transactions of the Clinical Society of London*. 7: 22–8.

Guy-Grand, B. and Goga, H. (1981), Conditioned salivation in obese subjects with different weight kinetics. *Appetite: Journal for Intake Research*. 2: 351–5.

Hagen, R.L. (1974), Group therapy versus bibliotherapy in weight reduction. *Behavior Therapy*. 5: 222–34.

Hall, B.D. and Smith, D.W. (1972), Prader-Willi syndrome. *Journal of Pediatrics*. 81 (2): 286–93.

Hall, J.C., Horne, K., O'Brien, P. and McWatts, J. (1983), Patient well-being after gastric bypass surgery for morbid obesity. *Australia and New Zealand Journal of Surgery*. 53: 321–4.

Hall, S.M., Hall, R.G., Borden, B.L., and Hanson, R.W. (1975), Follow-up strategies in the behavioural treatment of overweight. *Behaviour Research and Therapy*. 13: 167–72.

Hällström, T. and Noppa, H. (1981), Obesity in women in relation to mental illness, social factors and personality traits. *Journal of Psychosomatic Research*. 25 (2): 75–82.

Halmi, K., Eckert, E. and Falk, J. (1983), Cyproheptadine, an anti-depressant and weight-inducing drug for anorexia nervosa. *Psycho-pharmacology Bulletin*. 1: 103–5.

Halmi, K.D., Goldberg, S.C., Eckert, E., Casper, R. and Davis, J.M. (1977), Pretreatment evaluation in anorexia nervosa. *Anorexia Nervosa*. ed. R.A. Vigersky. New York, Raven Press. 43–54.

Halmi, K.A. and Falk, J.R. (1982), Anorexia nervosa. A study of outcome discriminators in exclusive dieters and bulimics. *Journal of the American Academy of Child Psychiatry*. 21 (4): 369–75.

Halmi, K.A., Falk, J.R. and Schwartz, E. (1981), Binge-eating and vomiting: a survey of a college population. *Psychological Medicine*. 11: 697–706.

Halmi, K.A., Long, M., Stunkard, A.J. and Mason, E. (1980), Psychiatric diagnosis of morbidly obese gastric by-pass patients. *American Journal of Psychiatry*. 137 (4): 470–2.

Halmi, K., Powers, P. and Cunningham, S. (1975). Treatment of anorexia nervosa with behaviour modification: effectiveness of formula feeding and isolation. *Archives of General Psychiatry*. 32: 93–6.

Halmi, K.A., Struss, A. and Goldberg, S.C. (1978), An investigation of weights in parents of anorexia nervosa patients. *Journal of Nervous and Mental Disease*. 166: 358–61.

Halmi, K.A., Stunkard, A.J. and Mason, E.E. (1980), Emotional responses to weight reduction by three methods: diet, jejunoileal bypass, and gastric bypass. *American Journal of Clinical Nutrition*. 33: 446–51.

Hamilton, M. (1960), A rating scale for depression. *Journal of Neurology, Neurosurgery and Psychiatry*. 23; 56–62.

Handen, B.L., Mandell, F. and Russo, D. (1986), Feeding induction in children who refuse to eat, *American Journal of Diseases in Children*. 140: 52–4.

HANES II. National Center for Health Studies. Plan and Operation of the National Health and Nutrition Examination Survey 1976–80. Washington D.C.: US Public Health Service 1981. DHSS Publication no. (PHS) 81–1317. (Vital and Health Statistics, series 1, no.15).

Hankin, J., Reed, D., Labarthe, D., Nichaman, M. and Stallones, R. (1970), Dietary and disease patterns among Micronesians. *American Journal of Clinical Nutrition*. 23: 346–57.

Hanna, C.F., Loro, A.D. and Power, D.D. (1981), Differences in the degree of overweight: a note on its importance. *Addictive Behaviors*. 6 (1): 61–2.

Hanson, R.D., Borden, B.L., Hall, S.M. and Hall, R.G. (1976). Use of programmed instruction in teaching self-management skills to overweight adults. *Behavior Therapy*. 7: 366–73.

Harmatz, M.G. and Lapuc, P. (1968), Behavior modification of overeating in a psychiatric population. *Journal of Consulting and Clinical Psychology*. 32: 583–7.

Harris, M.B. (1969), Self-directed programme for weight control: a pilot study. *Journal of Abnormal Psychology*. 74: 263–70.

Harris, M.B. (1983), Eating habits, restraint, knowledge and attitudes toward obesity. *International Journal of Obesity*. 7: 271–86.

Harris, M.B. and Bruner, C.G. (1971), A comparison of a self-control and a contract procedure for weight control. *Behaviour Research and Therapy*. 9: 347–54.

Harris, M.B., Sutton, M., Kaufman, E.M., and Carmichael, C.W. (1980), Correlates of success and retention in a multifaceted, long-term behavior modification program for obese adolescent girls. *Addictive Behaviors*. 5 (1): 25–34.

Harris, R.T. (1983), Bulimarexia and related serious eating disorders with medical complications. *Annals of Internal Medicine*. 99 (6): 800–7.

Hashim, S. and Van Itallie, T.B. (1965), Studies in normal and obese subjects with a monitored food dispensing device. *Annals of the New York Academy of Science*. 131 (Art 1): 654–61.

Hatsukami, D., Eckert, E., Mitchell, J.E. and Pyle, R. (1984), Affective disorder and substance abuse in women with bulimia. *Psychological Medicine*. 14: 701–4.

Haugh, R.M. and Markesbery, W.R. (1983), Hypothalamic astrocytoma. Syndrome of hyperphagia, obesity, and disturbances of behavior and endocrine and autonomic function. *Archives of Neurology*. 40 (9): 560–3.

Hawkins, C. (1976), Diseases of the alimentary system. Anorexia and loss of weight. *British Medical Journal*. 2 (6048): 1373–5.

Hawley, R.M. (1985), The outcome of anorexia nervosa in younger subjects. *British Journal of Psychiatry*. 146: 657–60.

Haynes, R.B. (1976), A critical review of the 'Determinants' of patient compliance with therapeutic regimens. *Compliance with Therapeutic Regimens*. ed. D.L. Sackett and R.B. Haynes. London and Baltimore, Johns Hopkins University Press. 26–39.

Heckerman, C.L. and Prochaska, J.O. (1976), Development and evaluation of weight reduction procedures in a health maintenance organisation. *Obesity, Behavioral Approaches to Dietary Management*. B.J. Williams, S. Martin and C.P. Foreyt. New York, Brunner Mazel. 215–28.

Heinzelmann, F. and Bagley, R.W. (1970), Response to physical activity programmes and their effects on Health Behaviour. *Public Health Reports*. 85: 905–11.

Held, M.L. and Snow, D.L. (1972), MMPI, I–E control, and Problem Check List scores of obese adolescent females. *Journal of Clinical Psychology*. 28 (4): 523–5.

Hendren, R.L. (1983), Depression in anorexia nervosa. *Journal of the American Academy for Child Psychiatry*. 22: 59–62.

Herman, C.P. and Mack, D (1975), Restrained and unrestrained eating. *Journal of Personality*. 43: 647–60.

Herman, C.P. and Polivy, J. (1975), Anxiety, restraint, and eating behaviour. *Journal of Abnormal Psychology*. 84 (6): 666–72.

Herman, C.P. and Polivy, J. (1980), Restrained eating. *Obesity*. ed. A.J. Stunkard. Philadelphia, W.B. Saunders. 208–25.

Herman, C.P., Polivy, J., Klajner, F. and Esses, V.M. (1981), Salivation in dieters and non-dieters. *Appetite*. 2 (4): 356–61.

Hernandez, L. and Hoebel, B.G. (1980), Basic mechanisms of feeding and weight regulation. *Obesity*. ed A.J. Stunkard. Philadelphia, W.B. Saunders. 25–47.

Heron, G. and Johnston, D. (1976), Hypothalamic tumor presenting as anorexia nervosa. *American Journal of Psychiatry*. 133: 580–2.

Herzog, D.B. (1984), Are anorexic and bulimic patients depressed? *American Journal of Psychiatry*. 141 (12): 1594–7.

Herzog, D.B. (1984a), Pharmacotherapy of anorexia nervosa and bulimia. *Pediatric Annals*. 13: 915–23.

Herzog, D.B. and Norman, D.K. (1985), Subtyping eating disorders. *Comprehensive Psychiatry* 26 (4): 375–80.

Hibscher, J.A. and Herman, C.P. (1977), Obesity, dieting, and the expression of 'obese' characteristics. *Journal of Comparative and Physiological Psychology*. 91: 374–80.

Hill, S.W. and McCutcheon, N.B. (1975), Eating responses of obese and non-obese humans during dinner meals. *Psychosomatic Medicine*. 37 (5): 395–401.

Hillard, J.R. and Hillard, P.J. (1984), Bulimia, anorexia nervosa, and diabetes: deadly combinations. *Psychiatric Clinics of North America*. 7 (2): 367–79.

Hodgson, R.J. and Greene, J.B. (1980), The saliva priming effect, eating speed and the measurement of hunger. *Behaviour Research and Therapy*. 18 (4): 243–47.

Holland, J.C.B., Rowland, J. and Plumb, M. (1977), Psychological aspects of anorexia in cancer patients. *Cancer Research*. 37 (7): 2425–8.

Holm, V.A. and Pipes, P.L. (1976), Food and children with Prader-Willi syndrome. *American Journal of Diseases in Childhood*. 130: 1063–7.

Homant, R.J. and Kennedy, D.B. (1982), Attitudes towards ex-offenders: a comparison of social stigmas. *Journal of Criminal Justice*. 10 (5): 383–91.

Hopkinson, G. and Bland, R.C. (1982), Depressive syndromes in grossly obese women. *Canadian Journal of Psychiatry*. 27 (3): 213–15.

Hoyenga, K.B. and Hoyenga, K.T. (1982), Gender and energy balance: sex differences in adaptation for feast and famine. *Physiology and Behavior*. 28 (3): 545–63.

Hsu, L.K. (1980), Outcome of anorexia nervosa: a review of the literature (1954 to 1978). *Archives of General Psychiatry*. 37 (9): 1041–6.

Hsu, L.K.G. (1982), Is there a body image disturbance in anorexia nervosa? *Journal of Nervous and Mental Disease* 5: 305–7.

Hsu, L.K. (1983), The aetiology of anorexia nervosa. *Psychological Medicine*. 13 (2): 231–8.

Hsu, L.K. and Liberman, S. (1982), Paradoxical intention in the treatment of chronic anorexia nervosa. *American Journal of Psychiatry*. 139 (5): 650–3.

Hudson, J.I., Pope, H.G., Jonas, J.M. and Yurgelun-Todd, D. (1983), Family history study of anorexia nervosa and bulimia. *British Journal of Psychiatry*. 142: 133–38.

Hudson, J.I., Wentworth, S.M., Hudson, M. and Pope, H.G. (1985), Prevalence of anorexia nervosa and bulimia among young adult diabetic women. *Journal of Clinical Psychiatry*. 46: 88–9.

Huon, G. and Brown, L.B. (1984), Psychological correlates of weight control among anorexia nervosa patients and normal girls. *British Journal of Medical Psychology*. 57: 61–6.

Huse, D.M. and Lucas, A.R. (1984), Dietary patterns in anorexia nervosa. *American Journal of Clinical Nutrition*. 40 (2): 251–4.

Igoin, L. and Apfelbaum, M. (1982), Differences in tolerance to frustration between moderately obese and severely obese subjects. *International Journal of Obesity*. 6: 227–32.

Israel, A.C., Stolmaker, L., Sharp, J.P., Silverman, W.K. and Simon, L.G.

(1984), An evaluation of two methods of parental involvement in treating obese children. *Behavior Therapy*. 15: 266–72.

Jackson, N.J. and Ormiston, L.H. (1977), Diet and weight control clinic: a status report. Stanford Heart Disease Prevention Program. Unpublished manuscript. Stanford University.

Jeffcoate, W.J., Laurance, B.M., Edwards, C.R.W. and Besser, G.M. (1980), Endocrine function in the Prader-Willi syndrome. *Clinical Endocrinology*. 12: 81–9.

Jeffery, R.W., Bjornson-Benson, W.M., Rosenthal, B.S., Kurth, C.L. and Dunn, M.M. (1984), Effectiveness of monetary contracts with two repayment schedules of weight reduction in men and women from self-referred and population samples. *Behavior Therapy*. 15 (3): 273–9.

Jeffery, R.W., Danaher, B.G., Killen, J., Farquhar, J.W. and Kinnier, R. (1982), Self-administered programs for health behavior change: smoking cessation and weight reduction by mail. *Addictive Behaviors*. 7: 57–63.

Jeffery, R.W., Thompson, P.D. and Wing, R.R. (1978a), Effects on weight reduction of strong monetary contracts for calorie restriction on weight loss. *Behaviour Research and Therapy*. 16 (5): 3–9.

Jeffery, R.W., Vender, M. and Wing, R. (1978), Weight loss and behavior change one year after behavioral treatment of obesity. *Journal of Consulting and Clinical Psychology*. 46 (2): 368–9

Jeffery, R.W., Wing, R.R. and Stunkard, A.J. (1978), Behavioral treatment of obesity: the state of the art 1976. *Behavior Therapy*. 9: 189–99.

Jeffrey, D.B. (1974), A comparison of the effects of external control and self-control on the modification and maintenance of weight. *Journal of Abnormal Psychology*. 83: 404–10.

Jeffrey, D.B. and Christensen, E.R. (1975), Behavior therapy versus willpower in the management of obesity. *The Journal of Psychology*. 90: 303–311.

Jeffrey, D.B., McLellarn, R.W. and Fox, D.T. (1982), The development of children's eating habits: the role of television commercials. *Health Education Quarterly*. 9 (2–3): 174–89.

Jennings, K.P. and Klidjian, A.M. (1974), Acute gastric dilatation in anorexia nervosa. *British Medical Journal*. 2: 477–8.

Jiang, C.L. and Hunt, J.N. (1983), The relation between freely chosen meals and body habitus. *American Journal of Clinical Nutrition*. 38: 32–40.

Johnson, C. and Berndt, D.J. (1983), Preliminary investigation of bulimia and life adjustment. *American Journal of Psychiatry*. 140 (6): 774–7.

Johnson, C.L., Stuckey, M.K., Lewis, L.D. and Schwartz, D.M. (1982), Bulimia: a descriptive survey of 316 cases. *International Journal of Eating Disorders*. 2:3–16.

Johnson, C.L., Stuckey, M., Lewis, L.D. and Schwartz, D.M. (1983), A survey of 509 cases of self-reported bulimia. *Anorexia Nervosa: Recent Developments*. ed. P.L. Darby, P.E. Garfinkel, D.M. Garner, D.Y. Coscina. New York, Alan R. Liss. 159–71.

Johnson, C.L., Stuckey, M. and Mitchell, J. (1983a), Pharmacological treatment of anorexia nervosa and bulimia: review and synthesis. *Journal of Nervous and Mental Diseases* 171(9): 524–34.

Johnson, D. and Larson, R. (1982), Bulimia: an analysis of moods and behavior. *Psychosomatic Medicine*. 44: 341–51.

Johnson, S.F., Swenson, W.M., Gastineau, C.F. (1976), Personality characteristics in obesity: relation of MMPI profile and age of onset of obesity to success in weight reduction. *American Journal of Clinical Nutrition*. 29 (6): 626–32.

Johnson-Sabine, E.C., Wood, K.H. and Wakeling, A. (1984), Mood changes in bulimia nervosa. *British Journal of Psychiatry*. 145: 512–16.

Johnston, J.G. and Robertson, W.O. (1977), Fatal ingestion of table salt by an adult. *Western Journal of Medicine*. 126: 141–3.

Jones, D.J., Fox, M.M., Babigian, H.M. and Hutton, H.E. (1980), Epidemiology of anorexia nervosa in Monroe County, New York: 1960–1976. *Psychosomatic Medicine*. 42 (6): 551–8.

Jordan, H.A., Canavan, A.J. and Steer, R.A. (1985), Patterns of weight change: the interval 6 to 10 years after initial weight loss in a cognitive – behavioral treatment program. *Psychological Reports* 57(1): 195–203.

Jung, R.T., Campbell, R.G., James, W.P. and Cullingham, B.A. (1982), Altered hypothalamic and sympathetic responses to hypoglycaemia in familial obesity. *Lancet* 1 (8280): 1043–6.

Kalucy, R.C., Crisp, A.H. and Harding, B. (1977), A study of 56 families with anorexia nervosa. *British Journal of Medical Psychology*. 50 (4): 381–95.

Kamalian, N., Keesey, R.E. and Zu Rhein, G.M. (1975), Lateral hypothalamic demyelination and cachexia in a case of 'malignant' multiple sclerosis. *Neurology*. 25: 25–30.

Kaplan, H.T. and Kaplan, H.S. (1957), The psychosomatic concept of obesity. *Journal of Nervous and Mental Disease*. 125: 181–201.

Kare, M.R. and Beauchamp, G.K. (1985), The role of taste in the infant diet. *American Journal of Clinical Nutrition*. 41: 418–22.

Katahn, M., Pleas, J., Thackrey, M. and Wallston, K.A. (1982), Relationship of eating and activity self-reports to follow-up weight maintenance in the massively obese. *Behavior Therapy*. 13 (4): 521–8.

Katz, J.L., Kuperberg, A., Pollack, C.P., Walsh, B.T., Zumoff, B., Weiner, H. (1984), Is there a relationship between eating disorder and affective disorder? New evidence from sleep recordings. *American Journal of Psychiatry*. 141 (6): 753–9.

Kauli, R., Prager-Lewin, R. and Laron, Z. (1978), Pubertal development in the Prader-Willi syndrome. *Acta Paediatrica Scandinavica*. 37: 763–7.

Keane, T.M., Geller, S.E. and Scheirer, C.J. (1981), A parametric investigation of eating styles in obese and non-obese children. *Behavior Therapy*. 12 (2): 280–6.

Keefe, P.H., Wyshogrod, D., Weinberger, E. and Agras, W.S. (1984), Binge eating and outcome of behavioural treatment of obesity: a preliminary report. *Behaviour Research and Therapy*. 22 (3): 319–21.

Keesey, R.E., Boyle, P.C., Kemnitz, J.W. and Mitchel, J.S. (1976), The role of the lateral hypothalamus in determining the body weight set point. *Hunger: Basic Mechanisms and Clinical Implications*. ed. D. Novin, W. Wyrwicka and G. Bray. New York, Raven Press. 243–55.

Keesey, R.E. and Corbett, S.W. (1984), Metabolic defence of the body weight set-point. *Eating and its Disorders*. ed. A.J. Stunkard and E. Stellar. New York, Raven Press. 87–96.

Keith, R.R. and Vandenberg, S.G. (1974), Relation between orality and weight. *Psychological Reports*. 35: 1205–6.

Kendell, R.E., Hall, D.J., Hailey, A. and Babigian, H.M. (1973), The epidemiology of anorexia nervosa. *Psychological Medicine*. 3: 200–3.

Kenny, F.T. and Solyom, L. (1971), The treatment of compulsive vomiting through faradic disruption of mental images. *Journal of the Canadian Medical Assocation*. 105: 1071–3.

Keys, A., Brozek, J., Henschel, A., Mickelson, O. and Taylor, H.L. (1950), *The Biology of Human Starvation*. Minneapolis: University of Minnesota Press.

King, S. (1983), Trends in meal planning and eating habits. *Food and People*. ed. M.R. Turner. British Nutrition Foundation, London, John Libbey. 43–65.

Kingsley, R.G. and Wilson, G.T. (1977), Behavioral therapy for obesity: a comparative investigation of long-term efficacy. *Journal of Consulting and Clinical Psychology*. 45: 288–98.

Kirkley, B.G., Schneider, J.A., Agras, W.S. and Bachman, J.A. (1955). A comparison of two group treatments for bulimia. *Journal of Consulting and Clinical Psychology*. 53(1): 43–8.

Kirschenbaum, D.S. and Flanery, R.C. (1983), Behavioral contracting: outcomes and elements. *Progress in Behavior Modification*. 15: 217–75.

Kirschenbaum, D.S., Stalonas, P.M., Zastowny, T.R. and Tomarken, A.J. (1985). Behavioural treatment of adult obesity: attentional controls and a two-year follow up. *Behaviour Research and Therapy* 23 (6): 675–82.

Klajner, F., Herman, C.P., Polivy, J. and Chhabra, R. (1981), Human obesity, dieting, and anticipatory salivation to food. *Physiology and Behavior*. 27 (2): 195–8.

Kleine, W. (1925), Periodische Schlafsucht. *Monatschrift für Psychiatrische Neurologie*. 57: 285–320.

Koch, U. and Gromus, B. (1983), Seven years of experience in treatment of obese patients with an interdisciplinary model: changes in weight and behavior. International Congress of Obesity in New York. Poster presentation.

Kornhaber, A. (1970). The stuffing syndrome. *Psychosomatics*. 11: 580–4.

Kral, J.G. (1983), Surgical therapy. *Contemporary Issues in Clinical Nutri-*

tion. 4. Obesity. ed. M.R.C. Greenwood. Edinburgh, Churchill Livingstone. 25–38.

Krantz, D.S. (1979), A naturalistic study of social influences on meal size among moderately obese and non-obese subjects. *Psychosomatic Medicine.* 41 (1): 19–27.

Krassner, H.A., Brownell, K.D. and Stunkard, A.J. (1979), Cleaning the plate: food left by overweight and normal weight persons. *Behaviour Research and Therapy.* 17 (2): 155–6.

Kron, L., Katz, J.L., Gorzynski, G. and Weiner, H. (1978), Hyperactivity in anorexia nervosa: a fundamental clinical feature. *Comprehensive Psychiatry.* 19 (5): 433–40.

Kulesza, W. (1982), Dietary intake in obese women. *Appetite.* 3 (1): 61–8.

Kurman, L. (1978), An analysis of messages concerning food, eating behaviours, and ideal body image on prime-time American network television. *Dissertation Abstract.*

Kyriakides, M., Silverstone, T., Jeffcoate, W. and Laurance, B. (1980), Effect of naloxone on hyperphagia in Prader-Willi syndrome. *Lancet.* April 19. 876–7.

Lacey, J.H. (1983), Bulimia nervosa, binge eating, and psychogenic vomiting: a controlled treatment study and longterm outcome. *British Medical Journal.* May 21, 286 (6378): 1609–13.

Lacey, J. and Crisp, A. (1980), Hunger, food-intake and weight: the impact of clomiprimine on a refeeding anorexia nervosa population. *Post Graduate Medical Journal.* 56. Suppl. 1: 79–85.

Lacey, J.H. and Gibson, E. (1985), Does laxative abuse control body weight? A comparative study of purging and vomiting bulimics. Human Nutrition: Applied Nutrition 39(1): 36–42.

Laurence, B.M., Brito, A. and Wilkinson, J. (1981), Prader-Willi syndrome after age fifteen years. *Archives of Diseases in Childhood.* 56 (3): 181–6.

Lavigne, J.V., Burns, W.J. and Cotter, P.D. (1981), Rumination in infancy: Recent behavioural approaches. *International Journal of Eating Disorders* 1(1): 70–82.

Lefcourt, H.M. (1976), *Locus of Control: Current Trends in Theory and Research.* Laurence Erlbaum Associated Publishers, New York, John Wiley.

Leitenberg, H., Agras, W.S., Thomson, L.E. (1968), A sequential analysis of the effect of selective positive reinforcement in modifying anorexia nervosa. *Behaviour Research and Therapy.* 6: 211–18.

Leon, G.R. (1975), Personality, body image, and eating pattern changes in overweight persons after weight loss. *Recent Advances in Obesity Research. 1.* ed. A. Howard. London, Newman. 228–38.

Leon, G.R. (1983), Anorexia nervosa: the question of treatment emphasis. *Perspectives on Behavior Therapy in the Eighties*, vol. 9. ed. M. Rosenbaum, C.M. Franks and Y. Jaffe. New York, Springer. Chap. 19: 363–77.

Leon, G.R. (1984), Anorexia nervosa and sports activities. *Behavior Therapist*. 7 (1): 9–10.

Leon, G.R. and Chamberlain, K. (1973), Comparison of daily eating habits and emotional states of overweight persons successful or unsuccessful in maintaining a weight loss. *Journal of Consulting and Clinical Psychology*. 41 (1): 108–15.

Lerner, R.M. and Gellert, E. (1969), Body build identification, preference and aversion in children. *Developmental Psychology*. 1: 456–62.

Levin, M. (1936), Periodic somnolence and morbid hunger: a new syndrome. *Brain*. 59: 494–504.

Levitt, H. and Fellner, C. (1965), MMPI profiles of three obesity subgroups. *Journal of Consulting Psychology*. 29: 11–16.

Levitz, L.S. and Stunkard, A.J. (1974), A therapeutic coalition for obesity: Behavior modification and patient self-help. *American Journal of Psychiatry*. 131: 423–7.

Ley, P. (1976), Toward better doctor-patient communication: contributions from experimental and social psychology. *Communications between Doctors and Patients*. ed. A.E. Bennett. London, Oxford University Press for the Nuffield Provincial Hospitals Trust.

Ley, P. (1980), Psychological, social and cultural determinants of acceptable fatness. *Nutrition and Lifestyles*. ed. M.R. Turner. London, Applied Science Publishers. 105–118.

Ley, P. (1984), Some tests of the hypothesis that obesity is a defence against depression. *Behaviour Research and Therapy*. 22 (2): 197–9.

Ley, P., Bradshaw, P.W., Kincey, J.A., Couper-Smartt, J. and Wilson, M. (1975), Psychological variables in the control of obesity. *Obesity*. ed. W.L. Burland, P. Samuel and S. Yudkin. Servier Research Institute Symposium, Edinburgh, Churchill Livingstone. 317–37.

Ley, P. and Spelman, M.S. (1967), *Communicating with the Patient*. London, Staples Press.

Linden, W. (1980), Multi-component behavior therapy in a case of compulsive binge-eating followed by vomiting. *Journal of Behavior Therapy and Experimental Psychiatry*. 11 (4): 297–300.

Linton, P.H., Conley, M., Kuechenmeister, C. and McCluskey, H. (1972), Satiety and obesity. *American Journal of Clinical Nutrition*. 368–70.

Long, C.G. and Cordle, C.J. (1982), Psychological treatment of binge-eating and self-induced vomiting. *British Journal of Medical Psychology*. 55: 139–45.

Loro, A.J. and Orleans, C.S. (1981), Binge eating in obesity: preliminary findings and guidelines for behavioral analysis and treatment. *Addictive Behaviors*. 6 (2): 155–66.

Lowe, M.R. and Fisher, E.B. Jr (1983), Emotional reactivity, emotional eating, and obesity: a naturalistic study. *Journal of Behavioral Medicine*. 6 (2): 135–49.

Lyketsos, G.C., Paterakis, P., Beis, A. and Lyketsos, C.G. (1985), Eating disorders in schizophrenia. *British Journal of Psychiatry*. 146: 255–61.

McAnarney, E.R., Greydanus, D.E., Camparella, V.A. and Hockelman, R.A. (1983), Rib fractures and anorexia nervosa. *Journal of Adolescent Health Care*. 4 (1): 40–3.

McCrea, C.W., Summerfield, A.B. and Rosen, B. (1982), Body image: a selective review of existing measurement techniques. *British Journal of Medical Psychology*. 55: 225–33.

McCrea, C. and Summerfield, A. (1983), Variable-image videoconfrontation as a method of assessing body-image distortion in the obese. International Congress on Obesity. New York. Poster presentation.

McGuffin, W.L. and Rogol, A.D. (1975), Response to LH – RH and clomiphene citrate in two women with the Prader-Labhart-Willi syndrome. *Journal of Clinical Endocrinology and Metabolism*. 41 (2): 325–31.

McKenna, R.J. (1972), Some effects of anxiety level and food cues on the eating behavior of obese and normal subjects: a comparison of the Schachterian and psychosomatic conceptions. *Journal of Personality and Social Psychology*. 22: 311–19.

McKenzie, J. (1980), Economic influences on food choice. *Nutrition and Lifestyles*. ed. M.R. Turner. London, Applied Science Publishers. 91–103.

Mackenzie, M. (1985), The anthropology of others and of ourselves related to the weanling. *American Journal of Clinical Nutrition*. 41: 497–501.

McReynolds, W.T. (1982), Towards a psychology of obesity: review of research on the role of personality and level of adjustment. *International Journal of Eating Disorders*. 2(1): 37–58.

McReynolds, W.T. and Lutz, R.N. (1974), Weight loss resulting from two behavior modification procedures with nutritionists as therapists. Paper read at Association for Advancement of Behavior Therapy, Chicago. Cited by Weiss (1977).

McReynolds, W.T., Lutz, R.N., Paulsen, B.K. and Kohrs, M.B. (1976), Weight loss from two behavior modification procedures with nutritionists as therapists. *Behavior Therapy*. (7): 283–91.

Maddox, G.L. (1968), Overweight as social deviance and disability. *Journal of Health and Social Behavior*. 9: 287–98.

Mahoney, M.J. (1974), Self-reward and self-monitoring techniques for weight control. *Behavior Therapy*. 5: 48–57.

Mahoney, M.J. and Mahoney, K. (1976), *Permanent Weight Control: A Total Solution to the Dieter's Dilemma*. New York, Norton.

Maiman, L.A. Wang, V.L., Becker, M.H., Finlay, J. and Simonson, M. (1979), Attitudes towards obesity and the obese among professionals. *Journal of the American Dietetic Association*. 74 (3): 331–6.

Maloney, M.J. and Farrell, M.K. (1980), Treatment of severe weight loss in anorexia nervosa with hyperalimentation and psychotherapy. *American Journal of Psychiatry*. 137 (3): 310–14.

Manno, B. and Marston, A.R. (1972), Weight reduction as a function of negative covert reinforcement versus positive covert reinforcement. *Behaviour Research and Therapy*. 10: 201–7.

Margo, J.L. (1985), Anorexia nervosa in adolescents. *British Journal of Medical Psychology* 58 (2): 193–5.

Marlatt, G.A. and Gordon, J.R. (1980), Determinants of relapse: implications for the maintenance of behavior change. *Behavioral Medicine: Changing Health Lifestyles*. ed. P. Davidson. New York, Brunner/Mazel. 410–52.

Marston, A.R. and Criss, J. (1984), Maintenance of successful weight loss: incidence and prediction. *International Journal of Obesity*. 8: 435–9.

Marwick, M.G. (1965), *Sorcery in its Social Setting*. Manchester University Press.

Mason, E.E., Printen, K.J., Blummers, T.J., Lewis, J.W. and Scott, D.H. (1980), Gastric by-pass in morbid obesity. *American Journal of Clinical Nutrition*. 33: 395–405.

Mazel, J. (1981), *The Beverley Hills Diet*. New York, Macmillan.

Meichenbaum, D. (1977), *Cognitive Behavior Modification*. New York, Plenum.

Mendelsohn, B.K. and White, R. (1982), Relation between body-esteem and self-esteem of obese and normal children. *Perceptual and Motor Skills*. 54 (3, pt 1): 899–905.

Metropolitan Life Insurance Company, New York (1960), Mortality among overweight men and women. *Statistical Bulletin*. 4: 1.

Meyers, A.W., Stunkard, A.J. and Coll, M. (1980), Food accessibility and food choice: test of Schachter's externality hypothesis. *Archives of General Psychiatry*. 37 (10): 1133–5.

Miles, S.W. and Wright, J.J. (1984), Psychoendocrine interaction in anorexia nervosa, and the retreat from puberty: a study of attitudes to adolescent conflict, and luteinising hormone response to luteinising hormone releasing factor in refed anorexia nervosa subjects. *British Journal of Medical Psychology*. 57: 49–56.

Miller, P.M. and Sims, K.L. (1981), Evaluation and component analysis of a comprehensive weight control program. *International Journal of Obesity*. 5: 57–65.

Mills, L. (1976), Amitriptyline therapy in anorexia nervosa. *Lancet*. ii. 687.

Mintz. S.W. (1982), Choice and occasion: sweet moments. *The Psychobiology of Food Selection*. ed. L.M. Barker. Westport, Connecticutt, Avi Publishing Co. 157–67.

Minuchin, S., Rosman, B.L. and Baker, L. (1978), *Psychosomatic Families: Anorexia Nervosa in Context*. Cambridge, Mass. and London, Harvard University Press.

Mitchell, C. and Stuart, R.B. (1984), Effect of self-efficacy on drop-out from obesity treatment. *Journal of Consulting and Clinical Psychology*. 52 (6): 1100–1.

Mitchell, J.E. and Goff, G. (1984), Bulimia in male patients. *Psychosomatics.* 25 (12): 909–13.

Mitchell, J.E. and Groat, R. (1984), A placebo-controlled, double-blind trial of amitriptyline in bulimia. *Journal of Clinical Psychopharmacology.* 4 (4): 186–93.

Mitchell, J.E., Pyle, R.L. and Eckert, E.D. (1981), Frequency and duration of binge-eating episodes in patients with bulimia. *American Journal of Psychiatry.* 138 (6): 835–6.

Moon, R.D. (1979), Monitoring human eating patterns during the ingestion of non-liquid foods. *International Journal of Obesity.* 3: 281–8.

Moore, D.C. (1977), Amitriptyline therapy in anorexia nervosa. *American Journal of Psychiatry.* 134: 1303–4.

Moore, M.D., Stunkard, A. and Srole, L. (1962), Obesity, social class and mental illness. *Journal of the American Medical Association.* 181: 962–6.

Morgan, H.G. and Russell, G.F.M. (1975), Value of family background and clinical features as predictors of long-term outcome in anorexia nervosa: 4 year follow-up study of 41 patients. *Psychological Medicine.* 5: 355–72.

Morley, J.E., Levine, A.S. and Rowland, N.E. (1983), Mini review. Stress induced eating. *Life Sciences.* 32 (19): 2169–82.

Morrison, S.D. (1976), Control of food intake in cancer cachexia: a challenge and a tool. *Physiology and Behavior.* 17: 705–14.

Morrison, S.D. (1978), Origins of anorexia in neoplastic disease. *American Journal of Clinical Nutrition.* 31 (6): 1104–7.

Mott, T. Jr and Roberts, J. (1979), Obesity and hypnosis: a review of the literature. *American Journal of Clinical Hypnosis.* 22 (1): 3–7.

Munoz, R.A. (1984), The basis for the diagnosis of anorexia nervosa. *Psychiatric Clinics of North America.* 7 (2): 215–21.

Munro, J.F. (1979), Clinical use of anti-obesity agents. *The Treatment of Obesity.* ed. J.F. Munro. Lancaster, MTP Press. 85–121.

Munro, J.F. and Ford, M.J. (1982), Drug treatment of obesity. In *Drugs and Appetite.* ed. T. Silverstone. London, Academic Press. 125–57.

Murphy, J.K., Williamson, D.A., Buxton, A.E., Moody, S.C., Absher, N. and Warner, M. (1982), The long-term effects of spouse involvement upon weight loss and maintenance. *Behavior Therapy.* 13: 681–93.

Murray, R.O. (1947), Recovery from starvation. *Lancet.* 252: 507–11.

Needlemen, H.L. and Waber, D. (1977), The use of amitriptyline in anorexia nervosa. *Anorexia Nervosa.* ed. R.A. Vigersky. New York, Raven Press, 356–62.

Nirenberg, T.D. and Miller, P.M. (1982), Salivation: an assessment of food craving? *Behaviour Research and Therapy.* 20 (4): 405–7.

Nisbett, R.E. (1972), Hunger, obesity, and the ventromedial hypothalamus. *Psychological Review.* 79: 433–53.

Nisbett, R.E. and Gurwitz, S.B. (1970), Weight, sex, and the eating behavior of human newborns. *Journal of Comparative and Physiological Psychology.* 73: 245.

Nisbett, R.E. and Storms, M.D. (1973), Cognitive and social determinants of food intake. *Thought and Feeling: Cognitive Alteration of Feeling States*. ed. H. London and R.E. Nisbett. Chicago, Aldine. 190–208.

Nylander, I. (1971), The feeling of being fat and dieting in a school population: epidemiologic interview investigation. *Acta Sociomedica Scandinavica* 3: 17–26.

Office of Population Censuses and Surveys (1981), *OPCS Monitor*. ref. ss 81/1.

O'Neil, P.M., Currey, H.S., Sexauer, J.D., Riddle, F.E. and Molony-Sinnott, V. (1980), Persistence at three-year followup of male-female differences in weight loss. Paper presented at International Congress on Obesity, Rome.

Orbach, S. (1978), *Fat is a Feminist Issue: the Anti-diet Guide to Weight Loss*. New York and London, Paddington Press.

Orbach, S. (1982), *Fat is a Feminist Issue II*. New York, Berkley Publishing Corporation.

Otto, P.L., Sulzbacher, S.I. and Worthington-Roberts, B.S. (1982), Sucrose-induced behavior changes of persons with Prader-Willi syndrome. *American Journal of Mental Deficiency*. 86: 335–41.

Page T.J., Stanley, A.E., Richman, G.S., Deal, R.M. and Iwata, B.A. (1983), Reduction of food theft and long term maintenance of weight-loss in a Prader-Willi adult. *Journal of Behavior Therapy and Experimental Psychiatry*. 14 (3): 261–8.

Pai, J. (1950), Hypersomnia syndromes. *British Medical Journal*. 1: 522–4.

Palgi, A., Miller, M., Greenberg, I., Bistrian, B. and Blackburn, G. (1983), Behavioral variables associated with prolonged weight loss maintenance. 4th Annual International Congress on Obesity, New York. Poster presentation.

Palmer, R.L. (1979), The dietary chaos syndrome: a useful new term? *British Journal of Medical Psychology*. 52 (2): 187–90.

Parham, E.S., King, S.L., Bedell, M.L. and Martesteck, S. (1986), Weight control content of women's magazines: bias and accuracy. *International Journal of Obesity*. 10: 19–27.

Paykel, E.S. (1977), Depression and appetite. *Journal of Psychosomatic Research*. 21 (5): 401–7.

Pearce, J.W., Le Bow, M.D. and Orchard, J. (1981), Role of spouse involvement in the behavioral treatment of overweight women. *Journal of Consulting and Clinical Psychology*. 49 (2): 236–44.

Peckham, C.S., Stark, O., Simonite, V. and Wolff, O.H. (1983), Prevalence of obesity in British children born in 1946 and 1958. *British Medical Journal*. 286 (6373): 1237–42.

Penick, S.B., Filion, R., Fox, S. and Stunkard, A.J. (1971), Behavior modification treatment of obesity. *Psychosomatic Medicine*. 33 (1): 49–55.

Perri, M.G., McAdoo, W.G., Sperak, P.A. and Newlin, D.B. (1984), Effect of a multicomponent maintenance program on long-term weight-loss. *Journal of Consulting and Clinical Psychology*. 52 (3): 480–1.

Perri, M.G., Shapiro, R.M., Ludwig, W.W., Twentyman, C.T. and McAdoo, W.G. (1984a), Maintenance strategies for the treatment of obesity: an evaluation of relapse prevention training and post-treatment contact by mail and telephone. *Journal of Consulting and Clinical Psychology*. 52 (3): 404–13.

Pertschuk, M.J., Forster, J., Buzby, G. and Mullen, J.L. (1981), The treatment of anorexia nervosa with total parenteral nutrition. *Biological Psychiatry*. 16 (6): 539–50.

Peterson, P.E., Jeffrey, D.B., Bridgwater, C.A. and Dawson, B. (1984), How pronutrition television programming affects children's dietary habits. *Developmental Psychology*. 20 (1): 55–63.

Pinkerton, P. (1983), Disturbances of eating patterns. *Topics in Paediatric Medicine*. ed. J.A. Dodge. London, Pitman. 65–75.

Pliner, P. (1982), The effects of mere exposure on liking for edible substances. *Appetite: Journal for Intake Research*. 3: 283–90.

Pliner, P., Polivy, J., Herman, C.P. and Zakalusny, I. (1980), Short-term intake of overweight individuals and normal weight dieters and non-dieters with and without choice among a variety of foods. *Appetite* 1: 203–13.

Plumb, M., Holland, J., Park, S., Dykstia, L. and Holmes, I. (1975), Depressive symptoms in patients with advanced cancer: a controlled assessment (Abstract). *Psychosomatic Medicine*. 36: 459.

Polivy, J. (1976), Perception of calories and regulation of intake in restrained and unrestrained subjects. *Addictive Behaviors:* 1: 237–4.

Polivy, J. and Herman, C.P. (1976), Clinical depression and weight change, a complex relation. *Journal of Abnormal Psychology*. 85(3): 338–40.

Polivy, J. and Herman, C.P. (1985), Dieting and bingeing: a causal analysis. *American Psychologist*. 40 (2): 193–201.

Pope, H.G. and Hudson, J.I. (1984), *New Hope for Binge-Eaters: Advances in the Understanding and Treatment of Bulimia*. New York, Harper & Row.

Pope, H.G., Hudson, J.I., Jonas, J.M. and Yurgelun-Todd, D. (1983), Bulimia treated with imipramine: a placebo-controlled double-blind study. *American Journal of Psychiatry*. 140: 554–58.

Pope, H.G., Hudson, M.D. and Jonas, J.M. (1986), Bulimia in men: a series of fifteen cases. *Journal of Nervous and Mental Disease*. 174(2): 117–19.

Pope, H.G., Hudson, J.I. and Jonas, J.M. (1983a), Antidepressant treatment of bulimia: preliminary experience and practical recommendations. *Journal of Clinical Psychopharmacology*. 3 (5): 274–81.

Pope, H.G., Jr, Hudson, J.I. and Yurgelun-Todd, D. (1984), Anorexia nervosa and bulimia among 300 suburban women shoppers. *American Journal of Psychiatry*. 141 (2): 292–4.

Porikos, K.P., Booth, G. and Van Itallie, T.B. (1977), Effects of covert nutritive dilution on the spontaneous food intake of obese individuals: a pilot study. *American Journal of Clinical Nutrition*. 30: 1638–44.

Porikos, K.P., Hesser, M.F. and Van Itallie, T.B. (1982), Caloric regulation in normal-weight men maintained on a palatable diet of conventional foods. *Physiology and Behavior*. 29 (2): 292–300.

Prader, A., Labhart, A. and Willi, H. (1956), Ein Syndrom von Adipositas; Kleinwuchs, Kryptorchismus, und Oligophrenic nach Myatonieartigem Zustand im Neugeborenalter (Abstract). *Schweizerische Medizinische Wochenschrift*. 86: 1260–1.

Pudel, V.E., Metzdorff, M. and Oetting, M.X. (1975), Zur Persoehnlichkeit Adipoeser in psychologischen Tests Unter Beruecksichtigung latent Fettsuechtiger. *Zeitschrift für Psychosomatische Medizin und Psychoanalyse*. 21: 345–50.

Pudel, V.E. and Oetting, M. (1977), Eating in the laboratory: behavioural aspects of the positive energy balance. *International Journal of Obesity*. 1(4): 369–86.

Pugliese, M.T., Lifshitz, F., Grad, G., Fort, P. and Marks-Katz, M. (1983), Fear of obesity: a cause of short stature and delayed puberty. *New England Journal of Medicine*. 309 (9): 513–18.

Pyle, R.L., Mitchell, J.E. and Eckert, E.D. (1981), Bulimia, a report of 34 cases. *Journal of Clinical Psychiatry*. 42 (2): 60–4.

Rachman, S. (1981), The primacy of affect: some theoretical implications. *Behaviour Research and Therapy*. 19: 279–90.

Rand, C. and Stunkard, A.J. (1978), Obesity and psychoanalysis. *American Journal of Psychiatry*. 135: 547–51.

Rand, C.S. and Stunkard, A.J. (1983), Obesity and psychoanalysis: treatment and four-year follow-up. *American Journal of Psychiatry*. 140 (9): 1140–4.

Rau, J.H. and Green, R.S. (1975), Compulsive eating: a neuropsychologic approach to certain eating disorders. *Comprehensive Psychiatry* 16 (3): 223–31.

Reynolds, C.F., Kupfer, D.J., Christiansen, C.L., Auchenbach, R.C., Brenner, R.P., Sewitch, D.E., Tasha, L.S. and Coble, P.A. (1984), Multiple sleep latency test findings in Kleine Levin syndrome. *Journal of Nervous and Mental Diseases*. 172 (1): 41–4.

Richardson, S.A., Hastorf, A.H., Goodman, N. and Dornbush, S.M. (1961), Cultural uniformity in reaction to physical disabilities. *American Sociological Review*. 26: 241–7.

Ringrose, C.A. (1979), The use of hypnosis as an adjunct to curb obesity. *Public Health*, London. 93 (4): 252–7.

Rivinus, T.M., Biederman, J., Herzog, D.B., Kemper, K., Harper, G.P., Harmatz, J.S. and Houseworth, S. (1984), Anorexia nervosa and affective disorders: a controlled family history study. *American Journal of Psychiatry*. 14 (11): 1414–18.

Robbins, T.W. and Fray, P.J. (1980), Stress-induced eating. *Appetite: Journal for Intake Research*. 1: 103–33.

Rodin, G.M., Daneman, D., Johnson, L.E., Kenshole, A. and Garfinkel, P. (1985), Anorexia nervosa and bulimia in female adolescents with insulin dependant diabetes mellitus: a systematic study. *Journal of Psychiatric Research* 19 (2–3): 381–4.

Rodin, J. (1981), Current status of the internal-external hypothesis for obesity: what went wrong? *American Psychologist*. 36 (4): 361–72.

Rodin, J., Bray, G.A., Atkinson, R.L., Dahms, W.T., Greenaway, F.L., Hamilton, K. and Molitch, M. (1977), Predictors of successful weight loss in an outpatient obesity clinic. *International Journal of Obesity*. 1: 79–87.

Rodin, J. and Slochower, J. (1976), Externality in the non-obese: effects of environmental responsiveness on weight. *Journal of Personality and Social Psychology*. 33: 338–44.

Rodin, J. and Spitzer, L.B. (1983), The effects of type of sugar ingested on subsequent eating behavior. Paper given at International Congress of Obesity, New York.

Rogers, J.C. and Snow, T. (1982). An assessment of the feeding behaviors of the institutionalised elderly. *American Journal of Occupational Therapy*. 36(6): 375–80.

Rolls, B.J., Rolls, E.T. and Rowe, E.A. (1982), The influence of variety on human food selection and intake. *The Psychobiology of Human Food Selection*. ed. L.M. Barker. Westport, Connecticut. Avi Publishing Co. 101–22.

Rolls, B.J., Rowe, E.A., Rolls, E.T., Kingston, B., Megson, A. and Gunary, R. (1981), Variety in a meal enhances food intake in man. *Physiology and Behavior*. 26: 215–21.

Rolls, B.J., Van Duijvenvoorde, P.M. and Rowe, E.A. (1983), Variety in the diet enhances intake in a meal and contributes to the development of obesity in the rat. *Physiology and Behavior*. 31: 21–7.

Rolls, E.T. and Rolls, B.J. (1982), Brain mechanisms involved in feeding. *The Psychobiology of Human Food Selection*. ed. L.M. Barker. Westport, Connecticut, Avi Publishing Co. 33–62.

Romanczyk, R.G. (1974), Self-monitoring in the treatment of obesity. Parameters of reactivity. *Behavior Therapy*. 5: 531–40.

Romanczyk, R.G., Tracey, D.A., Wilson, G.T. and Thorpe, G.L. (1973), Behavioural techniques in the treatment of obesity: a comparative analysis. *Behaviour Research and Therapy*. 11 (4): 629–40.

Rose, G.A. and Williams, R.T. (1961), Metabolic studies on large and small eaters. *British Journal of Nutrition*. 15: 1–9.

Rosen, L.W. (1980), Modification of secretive or ritualized eating behavior in anorexia nervosa. *Journal of Behavior Therapy and Experimental Psychiatry*. 11 (2): 101–4.

Rosen, J.C. 1981), Effects of low-calorie dieting and exposure to diet-prohibited food on appetite and anxiety. *Appetite: Journal for Intake Research*. 2: 366–9.

Rosen, J.C. (1981), Effects of low-calorie dieting and exposure to diet-exposure and response prevention. *Behavior Therapy*. 13: 117–24.

Rosenberg, P., Herishanu, Y. and Beilin, B. (1977), Increased appetite (bulimia) in Parkinson's disease. *Journal of the American Geriatric Society*. 25 (6): 277–8.

Rossiter, E.M. and Wilson, G.T. (1985), Cognitive restructuring and response prevention in the treatment of bulimia nervosa. *Behaviour Research and Therapy*. 23 (3): 349–59.

Rotter, J.B. (1966), Generalised expectancies for internal versus external control of reinforcement. *Psychology Monographs*. 80 (1): 609.

Rowland, N.E., Antelman, S.M. and Seymour, M. (1976), Stress-induced hyperphagia and obesity in rats: a possible model for understanding human obesity. *Science*. 191 (4224): 310–12.

Royal College of Physicians (1983), *Obesity: a Report of the Royal College of Physicians*. 17 (1): 3–58.

Rozin, P. (1976), Psychobiological and cultural determinants of food choice. *Appetite and Food Intake*. ed. T. Silverstone. Dahlem Konferenzen, Berlin. 285–312.

Rozin, P. (1982), Human food selection: the interaction of biology, culture and individual experience. *The Psychobiology of Human Food Selection*. ed. L.M. Barker. Westport, Connecticut, Avi Publishing Co. 225–54.

Rozin, P. and Fallon, A.E. (1981), The acquisition of likes and dislikes for foods. *Criteria of Food Acceptance*. ed. J. Solms and R.L. Hall. Zurich, Foster Verlag A.G. 35–48.

Ruderman, A.J. (1985), Dysphoric mood and overeating: a test of restraint theory's disinhibition hypothesis. *Journal of Abnormal Psychology*. 94 (1): 78–85.

Ruderman, A.J., Belzer, L.J. and Halperin, A. (1985), Restraint, anticipated consumption, and overeating. *Journal of Abnormal Psychology*. 94 (4): 547–55.

Ruderman, A.J. and Christensen, H. (1983), Restraint theory and its applicability to overweight individuals. *Journal of Abnormal Psychology*. 92 (2): 210–15.

Ruderman, A.J. and Wilson, G.T. (1979), Weight, restraint, cognitions and counterregulation. *Behaviour Research and Therapy*. 17 (6): 581–90.

Russell, G.F.M. (1970), Anorexia nervosa: its identity as an illness and its treatment. *Modern Trends in Psychological Medicine*. Vol. 2, ed. J.H. Price. London, Butterworth. 131–64.

Russell, G.F.M. (1977), The present status of anorexia nervosa. *Psychological Medicine*. 7 (3): 363–7.

Russell, G.F.M. (1979), Bulimia nervosa: an ominous variant of anorexia nervosa. *Psychological Medicine*. 9: 429–48.

Russell, G.F.M. (1981), The current treatment of anorexia nervosa. *British Journal of Psychiatry*. 138: 164–6.

Russell, G.F.M., Campbell, P.G. and Slade, P.D. (1975), Experimental studies on the nature of the psychological disorder in anorexia nervosa. *Psychoneuroendocrinology*. 1: 45–56.

Sahakian, B.J. (1982), The interaction of psychological and metabolic factors

BIBLIOGRAPHY

in the control of eating and obesity. *Human Nutrition: Applied Nutrition*. 36A: 262–71.

Sandifer, B.A. and Buchanan, W.L. (1983), Relationship between adherence and weight loss in a behavioral weight reduction program. *Behavior Therapy*. 14 (5): 682–8.

Schachter, S. (1968), Obesity and eating. *Science*. 161: 751–6.

Schachter, S., Goldman, R. and Gordon, A. (1968), Effects of fear, food deprivation and obesity on eating. *Journal of Personality and Social Psychology*. 10: 91–7.

Schachter, S. and Gross, L. (1968), Manipulated time and eating behavior. *Journal of Personality and Social Psychology*. 10: 98–106.

Schiebel, D. and Castelnuovo-Tedesco, P. (1977), Studies of super-obesity III: body image changes after jejuno-ileal bypass surgery. *International Journal of Psychiatry in Medicine*. 8 (2): 117–23.

Schneider, J.A. and Agras, W.S. (1985), A cognitive behavioural group treatment of bulimia. *British Journal of Psychiatry*. 146: 66–9.

Schwartz, D.M. and Thompson, M.G. (1981), Do anorectics get well? Current research and future needs. *American Journal of Psychiatry*. 138 (3): 319–23.

Schwartz, R.S., Brunzell, J.D. and Bierman, E.L. (1981), Elevated adipose tissue lipoprotein lipase in the pathogenesis of obesity in Prader-Willi syndrome. *Prader-Willi Syndrome*. ed. V.A. Holm, S.J. Sulzbacher and P.L. Pipes. Baltimore, University Park Press. 137–43.

Sclafani, A. and Springer, D. (1976), Dietary obesity in adult rats: similarities to hypothalamic and human obesity syndromes. *Physiology and Behavior*. 17: 461–71.

Selvini-Palazzoli, M. (1978), *Self-starvation: From Individual to Family Therapy in the Treatment of Anorexia Nervosa*. trans. Arnold Pomeranz, c. 1974. New York, Jason Aronson.

Selvini-Palazzoli, M., Boscolo, C., Cecchin, G. and Prata, G. (1980), Hypothesizing – circularity – neutrality: three guidelines for the conductor of the session. *Family Process*. 19: 3–12.

Shields, J. (1962), *Monozygotic twins brought up apart and together: an investigation into the genetic and emotional causes of variation in personality*. London, Oxford University Press.

Shils, M.E. (1979), Nutritional problems induced by cancer. *Medical Clinics of North America*. 63 (5): 1009–25.

Shipman, W.G. and Plesset, M.R. (1963), Anxiety and depression in obese dieters. *Archives of General Psychiatry*. 8: 530–5.

Silverstone, J.T. (1968), Obesity. *Proceedings of the Royal Society of Medicine*. 61 (4): 371–5.

Silverstone, J.T. and Cooper, R.M. (1972), Short-term weight loss in refractory obesity. *Journal of Psychosomatic Research*, 16 (2): 123–8.

Silverstone, J.T., Gordin, R.P. and Stunkard, A.J. (1969), Social factors in obesity in London. *Practitioner*. 202: 682.

227

Simoons, F.J. (1982), Geography and genetics as factors. *The Psychobiology of Human Food Selection*. ed. L.M. Barker. Westport, Connecticut, Avi Publishing Co. 205–24.

Simopoulos, A.P. (1985), The health implications of overweight and obesity. *Nutrition Reviews*. 43 (2): 33–40.

Skilbeck, C.E., Tulips, J.G. and Ley, P. (1977), The effects of fear arousal, fear position, fear exposure and sidedness on compliance with dietary instructions. *European Journal of Social Psychiatry*. 7(2): 221–39.

Slade, P.D. (1973), A short anorexic behaviour scale. *British Journal of Psychiatry*. 122: 83–5.

Slade, P.D. (1982), Towards a functional analysis of anorexia nervosa and bulmia nervosa. *British Journal of Clinical Psychology*. 21 (3): 167–79.

Slade, P.D. and Russell, G.F. (1973), Experimental investigations of bodily perception in anorexia nervosa and obesity. *Psychotherapy and Psychosomatics*. 22 (2–6): 359–63.

Slochower, J. (1976), Emotional labeling and overeating in obese and normal weight individuals. *Journal of Psychosomatic Medicine*. 38 (2): 131–9.

Slochower, J.A. (1983), *Excessive Eating*, New York, Human Sciences Press. *Center for Policy Research Monograph Series*. ed. A. Etzioni.

Slochower, J. and Kaplan, S.P. (1980), Anxiety, perceived control and eating in obese and normal weight persons. *Appetite*. 1: 75–83.

Slochower, J., Kaplan, S.P. and Mann, L. (1981), The effects of life stress and weight on mood and eating. *Appetite*. 2: 115–25.

Smith, G.P. (1982), The physiology of the meal. *Drugs and Appetite*. ed. T. Silverstone. London, New York, Academic Press. 1–22.

Smith, G.R. and Medlik, L. (1983), Modification of binge-eating in anorexia nervosa: a single-case report. *Behavioural Psychotherapy*. 11 (3): 240–56.

Smith, N.J. (1980), Excessive weight loss and food aversion in athletes simulating anorexia nervosa. *Paediatrics*. 66: 139–42.

Snaith, R.P., Bridge, G.W.K. and Hamilton, M. (1976), The Leeds scales for the self-assessment of anxiety and depression. *British Journal of Psychiatry*. 128: 156–65.

Solyom, L., Freeman, R.J. and Miles, J.E. (1982), A comparative psychometric study of anorexia nervosa and obsessional neurosis. *Canadian Journal of Psychiatry*. 27 (4): 282–6.

Speaker, J., Schultz, C., Grinker, J.A. and Stern, J.S. (1983), Body size estimation and locus of control in obese adolescent boys undergoing weight reduction. *International Journal of Obesity*. 7: 73–83.

Spencer, J.A. and Fremouw, W.J. (1979), Binge-eating as a function of weight and restraint classification. *Journal of Abnormal Psychology*. 88: 262–7.

Spiegel, T.A. (1973), Caloric regulation of food intake in man. *Journal of Comparative Physiology and Psychology*. 84: 24–37.

Spitzer, L. and Rodin, J. (1981), Human eating behavior: a critical review of studies in normal weight and overweight individuals. *Appetite: Journal for Intake Research*. 2: 293–329.

Staffieri, J.R. (1967), A study of social stereotype of body image in children. *Journal of Personality and Social Psychology*. 7: 101–4.

Stalling, R.B. and Friedman, L. (1981), External social cues and obesity: the influence of others' food evaluations on eating. *Obesity and Metabolism*. 1 (2): 111–18.

Stalonas, P.M. Jr, Johnson, W.G. and Christ, M. (1978), Behavior modification for obesity: the evaluation of exercise, contingency management, and program adherence. *Journal of Consulting and Clinical Psychology*. 46 (3): 463–9.

Stalonas, P.M. and Kirschenbaum, D.S. (1985), Behavioral treatments for obesity: eating habits revisited. *Behavior Therapy*. 16: 1–14.

Stangler, R.S. and Printz, A.M. (1980), DSM III. Psychiatric diagnosis in a university population. *American Journal of Psychiatry*. 137: 937–40.

Stanton, B.R. and Exton-Smith, A.N. (1970), *A Longitudinal Study of the Dietary Habits of Elderly Women*. London, King Edward's Hospital Fund.

Stein, G.S., Hartshorn, J., Jones, J. and Steinberg, M. (1982), Lithium in a case of severe anorexia nervosa. *British Journal of Psychiatry*. 140: 526–8.

Steinberg, C.L. and Birk, J.M. (1983), Weight and compliance: male-female differences. *Journal of General Psychology*. 109: 95–102.

Steinhausen, H.C. and Glanville, K. (1983), A long-term follow-up of adolescent anorexia nervosa. *Acta Psychiatrica Scandinavica*. 68 (1): 1–10.

Stellar, E. (1984), Neural Basis: Introduction. *Eating and its Disorders*. ed. A.J. Stunkard and E. Stellar. New York, Raven Press. 1–4.

Stern, S.L., Dixon, K.N., Neruzer, E., Lake, M.D., Sansome, R.A., Smelzer, D.J., Lantz, S. and Schrier, S. (1984), Affective disorder in the families of women with normal weight bulimia. *American Journal of Psychiatry*. 141 (10): 1224–7.

Stewart, J.W., Walsh, B.T., Wright, L., Roose, S.R. and Glassman, A.H. (1984), An open trial of MAO inhibitors in bulimia. *Journal of Clinical Psychiatry*. 45: 217–19.

Stifler, L.T.P. (1983), Use of the protein sparing fast with an educational/behavioral program to manage the high risk obese patient. Paper presented at 4th International Congress on Obesity in New York.

Storz, N.S. (1982), Body image of obese adolescent girls in a high school and clinical setting. *Adolescence*. 17 (67): 667–72.

Strober, M., Goldenberg, I., Green, J. and Saxon, J. (1979), Body image disturbance in anorexia nervosa during the acute and recuperative phase. *Psychological Medicine*. 9: 695–701.

Strober, M., Morrell, W., Burroughs, J., Salkin, B. and Jacobs, C. (1985), A controlled family study of anorexia nervosa. *Journal of Psychiatric Research* 19 (2–3): 239–46.

Strober, M., Salkin, B., Burroughs, J. and Morrell, W. (1982), Validity of the bulimia-restricter distinction in anorexia nervosa: parental personality characteristics and family psychiatric morbidity. *Journal of Nervous and Mental Disease*. 170 (6): 345–51.

Stuart, R.B. (1967), Behavioural control of overeating. *Behaviour Research and Therapy*. 5: 357–65.

Stuart, R.B. (1980), Weight loss and beyond: are they taking it off and keeping it off? *Behavioral Medicine: Changing Lifestyles*. ed. P.O. Davidson and S.M. Davidson. New York, Brunner/Mazel. 151–94.

Stuart, R.B. and Davis, B. (1972), *Slim Chance in a Fat World: Behavioral Control of Obesity*. Champaign, Illinois, Research Press.

Stunkard, A.J. (1959), Eating patterns and obesity. *Psychiatric Quarterly*. 33: 284–95.

Stunkard, A.J. (1972), New therapies for the eating disorders. *Archives of General Psychiatry*. 26: 391–8.

Stunkard, A.J., d'Aquili, E., Fox, S. and Filion, R.D.L. (1972), Influences of social class on obesity and thinness in children. *Journal of the American Medical Association*. 221: 579–84.

Stunkard, A.J. and Brownell, K.D. (1980), Work-site treatment for obesity. *American Journal of Psychiatry*. 137 (2): 252–3.

Stunkard, A.J., Coll, M., Lundquist, S. and Meyers, A. (1980), Obesity and eating style. *Archives of General Psychiatry*. 37: 1127–9.

Stunkard, A.J., Craighead, L.W. and O'Brien, R. (1980), Controlled trial of behaviour therapy, pharmacotherapy, and their combination in the treatment of obesity. *Lancet* Nov. 15, 1045–7.

Stunkard, A.J. and Mazer, A. (1978), Smorgasbord and obesity. *Psychosomatic Medicine*. 40 (2): 173–5.

Stunkard, A.J. and Messick, S. (1985), The three-factor eating questionnaire to measure dietary restraint, disinhibition and hunger. *Journal of Psychosomatic Research*. 29 (1): 71–83.

Stunkard, A.J. and Penick, S.B. (1979), Behavior modification in the treatment of obesity. The problem of maintaining weight loss. *Archives of General Psychiatry*. 36 (7): 801–6.

Stunkard, A.J. and Rush, J. (1974), Dieting and depression re-examined: a critical review of reports of untoward responses during weight reduction for obesity. *Annals of Internal Medicine*. 81: 526–33.

Stunkard, A.J., Sorenson, T.I.A., Harris, C., Teasdale, T.W., Chakraborty, R., Schull, W.J. and Schulsinger, F. (1986), An adoption study of human obesity. *New England Journal of Medicine*. 314 (4): 193–8.

Swanson, D.W. and Dinello, F.A. (1970), Follow-up of patients starved for obesity. *Psychosomatic Medicine*. 32: 209–14.

Swift, W.J. (1982), The long-term outcome of early onset anorexia nervosa: a critical review. *Journal of the American Academy of Child Psychiatry*. 21 (1): 38–46.

Szmukler, G. (1982), Drug treatment of anorexic states. *Drugs and Appetite*. ed. T. Silverstone. London, Academic Press. 159–81.

Szmukler, G.I. (1983), A study of family therapy in anorexia nervosa: some methodological issues. *Anorexia Nervosa: Recent Developments in Research*. ed. P.L. Darby, P.E. Garfinkel, D.M. Garner and D.V. Coscina.

New York, Alan Liss. 417–26.

Szmukler, G.I., Eisler, I., Gillies, C. and Hayward, M.E. (1985), The implications of anorexia nervosa in a ballet school. *Journal of Psychiatric Research* 19 (2–3): 177–81.

Szmukler, G.I. and Russell, G.F.M. (1983), Diabetes mellitus, anorexia nervosa, and bulimia. *British Journal of Psychiatry*. 142: 305–8.

Szmukler, G.I. and Tantam, D. (1984), Anorexia nervosa: starvation dependence. *British Journal of Medical Psychology*. 57: 303–10.

Takram, C. and Cronin, D. (1976), Kleine-Levin syndrome in a female patient. *Canadian Psychiatric Association*. 21: 315–18.

Theander, S. (1970), Anorexia nervosa: a psychiatric investigation of 94 female cases. *Acta Psychiatrica Scandinavica*. Supplement 214.

Thomas, J.P. and Szmukler, G.I. (1985), Anorexia nervosa in patients of Afro-Caribbean extraction. *British Journal of Psychiatry*. 146: 653–6.

Thompson, D.A., Moskowitz, H.R. and Campbell, R.G. (1976), Effects of body weight and food intake on pleasantness ratings for a sweet stimulus. *Journal of Applied Physiology*. 41: 77–83.

Thompson, M.G. and Schwartz, D.M. (1982), Life-adjustment of women with anorexia nervosa and anorexic-like behavior. *International Journal of the Eating Disorders*. 1 (2): 48–60.

Tobias, L.C. and MacDonald, M.L. (1977), Internal locus of control and weight loss: an insufficient condition. *Journal of Consulting and Clinical Psychology*. 45: 647.

Tolstrup, K., Brinch, M., Isager, T., Nielsen, S., Nystrup, J., Severin, B. and Olesen, N.S. (1985), Long-term outcome of 151 cases of anorexia nervosa. *Acta Psychiatrica Scandinavica*. 71: 380–7.

Touyz, S.W., Beumont, P.J.V., Collins, J.K.P., McCabe, M. and Jupp, J. (1984), Body shape perception and its disturbance in anorexia nervosa. *British Journal of Psychiatry*. 144: 167–71.

Trenchard, E., Silverstone, T. and Laurance, B. (1986), in preparation.

Ureda, J.R. (1980), The effect of contract witnessing on motivation and weight loss in a weight control program. *Health Education Quarterly*. 7 (3): 163–85.

Vandereycken, W. and Pierloot, R. (1983), Drop-out during in-patient treatment of anorexia nervosa: a clinical study of 133 patients. *British Journal of Medical Psychology*. 56 (2): 145–56.

Vandereycken, W. and Van den Broucke, S. (1984), Anorexia nervosa in males: a comparative study of 107 cases reported in the literature (1970 to 1980). *Acta Psychiatrica Scandinavica*. 70: 447–54.

Van Itallie, T.B. and Vanderweele, D.A. (1981), The phenomenon of satiety. *Recent Advances in Obesity Research* III. ed. P. Björntorp, M. Cairella and A.N. Howard. London, John Libbey. 278–89.

Vaughn, C.E. and Leff, J.P. (1976). The influence of family and social factors on the course of a psychiatric illness: a comparison of schizophrenic and depressed neurotic patients. *British Journal of Psychiatry*. 129: 125–37.

BIBLIOGRAPHY

Vigersky, R.A. and Loriaux, D.L. (1977), The effect of cyproheptadine in anorexia nervosa: a double-blind trial. *Anorexia Nervosa*. ed. R. Vigersky. New York, Raven Press.

Vincent, J.P., Schiavo, L. and Nathan, R. (1976), Effect of deposit contracts and distractability on weight loss and maintenance. *Obesity: Behavioral Approaches to Dietary Management*. ed. B.J. Williams, S. Martin and J.P. Foreyt. New York, Brunner/Maazel. 65–97.

Wadden, T.A. and Flaxman, J. (1981), Hypnosis and weight loss: a preliminary study. *International Journal of Clinical and Experimental Hypnosis*. 19 (2): 162–73.

Wadden, T.A. and Stunkard, A.J. (1985), Social and psychological consequences of obesity. *Annals of Internal Medicine*, 103 (6 pt 2): 1062–7.

Wadden, T.A., Stunkard, A.J., Brownell, K.D. and Day, S.C. (1984), Treatment of obesity by behavior therapy and very low calorie diet: a pilot investigation. *Journal of Consulting and Clinical Psychology*. 52 (4): 692–4.

Waller, D.A., Janiel, S., Erman, M. and Emslie, G. (1984), Recognising and managing the adolescent with Kleine-Levin syndrome. *Journal of Adolescent Health Care*. 5 (2): 139–41.

Walsh, B.T., Stewart, J.W., Roose, S.P., Gladis, M. and Glassman, A.H. (1984), Treatment of bulimia with phenelzine: a double-blind, placebo-controlled, study. *Archives of General Psychiatry*. 41: 1105–9.

Walsh, B.T., Stewart, J.W., Wright, L., Harrison, W., Roose, S.P. and Glassman, A. (1982), Treatment of bulimia with monoamine oxidase inhibitors. *American Journal of Psychiatry*. 139 (12): 1629–30.

Wardle, J. (1980), Dietary restraint and binge eating. *Behavioral Analysis and Modification*. 4: 201–9.

Weinstein, L.B. (1981), Eating and socialising: activities of the elderly. *Activities, Adaptation and Aging*. 2 (1): 31–8.

Weiss, A.R. (1977), Characteristics of successful weight reducers: a brief review of predictor variables. *Addictive Behaviors*. 2 (4): 193–201.

Weiss, S.R. and Ebert, M.H. (1983), Psychological and behavioral characteristics of normal-weight bulimics and normal-weight controls. *Psychosomatic Medicine*. 45 (4): 293–303.

Welch, G.J. (1979), The treatment of compulsive vomiting and obsessive thoughts through graduated response delay, response prevention, and cognitive correction. *Journal of Behavior Therapy and Experimental Psychiatry*. 10: 77–82.

Wermuth, B.M., Davis, K.L., Hollister, L.E.E. and Stunkard, A.J. (1977), Phenytoin treatment of the binge-eating syndrome. *American Journal of Psychiatry*. 134: 1249–53.

White, J.H., Kelly, P. and Dorman, L. (1977), Clinical picture of atypical anorexia nervosa associated with hypothalamic tumors. *American Journal of Psychiatry*. 134 (3): 323–5.

Widdowson, E.M. (1936), A study of English diets by the individual method. Part I. *Mental Journal of Hygiene*. 36: 269–92.

232

Wijesinghe, B. (1973), Massed electrical aversion treatment of compulsive eating. *Journal of Behavior Therapy and Experimental Psychiatry*. 4: 133–5.

Wilson, C.A. (1982–3), The fear of being fat and anorexia nervosa. *International Journal of Psychoanalysis and Psychotherapy*. 9: 233–55.

Wilson, G.T. (1976), Obesity, binge eating and behavior therapy. *Behavior Therapy*. 7: 700–1.

Wilson, G.T. and Brownell, K. (1978), Behavior therapy for obesity: including family members in the treatment process. *Behavior Therapy*. 9: 943–5.

Wilson, G.T. and Brownell, K.D. (1980), Behavior therapy for obesity: and evaluation of treatment 'outcome'. *Advances in Behavior Research and Therapy*. 3: 49–86.

Wilson, G.T., Rossiter, E., Kleifield, E.I. and Lindholm, L. (1986), Cognitive-behavioral treatment of bulimia nervosa: a controlled evaluation. *Behaviour Research and Therapy*. 24(3): 277–88.

Wing, R.R., Epstein, L.H., Marcus, M.D. and Kupfer, D.J. (1984), Mood changes in behavioral weight loss programs. *Journal of Psychosomatic Research*. 28 (3): 189–96.

Wing, R.R., Epstein, L.H., Shapira, B. and Koeske, R. (1984a), Contingent therapist contact in a behavioral weight control program. *Journal of Consulting and Clinical Psychology*. 52 (4): 710–11.

Wing, R.R., Epstein, L.H., Marcus, M.D. and Koeske, R. (1984b), Intermittent low-calorie regimen and booster sessions in the treatment of obesity. *Behavior Research and Therapy*. 22 (4): 445–9.

Wing, R.R. and Jeffery, R.W. (1979), Outpatient treatments of obesity: a comparison of methodology and clinical results. *International Journal of Obesity*. 3: 261–79.

Winokur, A., March, V. and Mendels, J. (1980), Primary affective disorder in relatives of patients with anorexia nervosa. *American Journal of Psychiatry*. 137: 695–8.

Witherly, S.A., Pangborn, R.M. and Stern, J.S. (1980), Gustatory responses and eating duration of obese and lean adults. *Appetite: Journal for Intake Research*. 1: 53–63.

Wolf, E.M. and Crowther, J.H. (1983), Personality and eating habit variables as predictors of severity of binge eating and weight. *Addictive Behaviors*. 8 (4): 335–44.

Wollersheim, J.P., (1970), Effectiveness of group therapy based upon learning principles in the treatment of overweight women. *Journal of Abnormal Psychology*. 76: 462–74.

Wooley, O.W. and Wooley, S.C. (1975), The experimental psychology of obesity. *Obesity: Pathogenesis and Management*. ed. T. Silverstone. Acton, Massachusetts, Publishing Sciences Group.

Wooley, O.W. and Wooley, S. (1982), The Beverly Hills Eating Disorder: the mass marketing of anorexia nervosa. *International Journal of Eating*

Disorders. 1 (3): 58–69.

Wooley, O.W., Wooley, S.C. and Dunham, R.B. (1972), Calories and sweet taste: effects on sucrose preference in the obese and non-obese. *Physiology and Behaviour*. 9: 765–8.

Wooley, S.C. (1972), Physiologic versus cognitive factors in short-term regulation in the obese and non-obese. *Psychosomatic Medicine*. 34: 62–8.

Wooley, S.C. and Wooley, O.W. (1973), Salivation to the sight of food: a new measure of appetite. *Psychosomatic Medicine*. 35: 136–42.

Wooley, S. and Wooley, O. (1979), Obesity and women -1. A closer look at the facts. *Women's Studies International Quarterly*. 2: 69–79.

Wooley, S.C. and Wooley, O.W. (1980), Eating disorders: obesity and anorexia: *Women and Psychotherapy: An Assessment of Research and Practice*. ed. A. Brodsky, R. Hare-Mustin. New York, Guildford Press. 135–58.

Wooley, S.C. and Wooley, O.W. (1984), Should obesity be treated at all? *Research Publications of the Association of Research into Nervous and Mental Disease*. 62: 185–92.

Wooley, S.C., Wooley, O.W. and Dyrenforth, S.R. (1979), Obesity treatment re-examined: the case for a more tentative and experimental approach. *National Institute for Drug Abuse Research, Monograph*. 25: 238–50.

Wooley, S.C., Wooley, O.W. and Dyrenforth, S.R. (1980), The case against radical interventions. *American Journal of Clinical Nutrition*. 33: 465–71.

Wyrwicka, W. (1984), Anorexia nervosa as a case of complex instrumental conditioning. *Experimental Neurology*. 84: 579–89.

Yates, A., Leckey, K. and Shisslak, C.M. (1983), Running – an analogue of anorexia? *New England Journal of Medicine*. 308 (5): 251–5.

Yates, A.J. and Sambrailo, F. (1984), Bulimia nervosa: a descriptive and therapeutic study. *Behaviour Research and Therapy*. 22 (5): 503–17.

Yellowlees, A.J. (1985), Anorexia and bulimia in anorexia nervosa: a study of psychosocial functioning and associated psychiatric symptomatology. *British Journal of Psychiatry*. 146: 648–52.

Author Index

Subject Index

241

SUBJECT INDEX